The Dog Diet

THE
Dog Diet

A MEMOIR

What My Dog Taught Me
About Shedding Pounds, Licking Stress
and Getting a New Leash on Life

PATTI LAWSON

Health Communications, Inc.
Deerfield Beach, Florida

www.hcibooks.com

Library of Congress Cataloging-in-Publication Data

Lawson, Patti
    The dog diet : what my dog taught me about shedding pounds, licking
stress, and getting a new leash on life / Patti Lawson
        p. cm.
    ISBN 0-7573-0394-3
    1. Dogs—South Carolina—Charleston—Anecdotes. 2. Dogs—South
Carolina—Charleston—Humor. 3. Dog owners—South Carolina—
Charleston—Anecdotes. 4. Dogs—Food—Recipes. 5. Lawson, Patti. I. Title.

SF426.2.L39 2006
636.7'085—dc22

                                                                    2005055020

©2006 Patti Lawson
ISBN 0-7573-0394-3

Publisher: Health Communications, Inc.
             3201 S.W. 15th Street
             Deerfield Beach, FL 33442-8190

Cover design by Larissa Hise Henoch
Inside book design by Lawna Patterson Oldfield
Illustrations by David Voisard

To my wonderful dog, Sadie,
and to
Betty Wilson, who brought
Sadie into my life.

CONTENTS

*Part Two: Licking Stress and Getting a
            New Leash on Life*

Part Three: The Dog Diet Plan

ACKNOWLEDGMENTS

To these people I offer my greatest thanks:

Rodney, my rock, and the best "dad" Sadie could ever have.

My fantastic agent, Barbara Ellis, and the Scribes Literary Agency. She loved my project as much as I did and worked tirelessly to get it out there.

My editor, Elisabeth Rinaldi, whose dog Luna made it possible for her to understand my book from the very beginning. You were the editor from heaven!

My wonderful publicists, Kim Weiss at HCI and Rose Carrano in New York City. Thank you both for tolerating all my million marketing ideas and working so hard to get my book out to the world.

My publisher, HCI, you were my soul mate on this project.

My best friend, critic, editor, fellow lawyer, traveling sidekick and cheerleader, Season Atkinson. You are invaluable.

Patrick Grace and the Life Writing Class in Charleston, West Virginia. Your encouragement and support made *The Dog Diet* go from an idea to reality.

Judy Katz, Katz Creative, New York City. Your enthusiasm, knowledge and faith in my book are phenomenal.

Gina Crisp, who became my friend through the writing of this book and whose lovely mountain cabin provided the perfect place for me to write.

My secretary, Pam Rudiger. Without your assistance I could never have gotten everything done.

Doug Imbrogno and the *Charleston Gazette*. You gave me a chance by publishing my first travel story and making my column become a reality.

Mark Shaw and the Books for Life Foundation, Aspen, Colorado. Your guidance and advice were priceless.

Karin Vingle-Fuller, fellow columnist, friend and supporter. Thanks for all the inspiration.

Shelby Sharps, steadfast friend, who told me for years I should be "writing that down."

All the fantastic people I met and learned from at writing conferences, including Tim Bete, Craig Wilson, Michael Larsen and Dave Lieber.

Julie Anne Parks and Lynn Chandler Willis of the Triad Writers Workshop, Greensboro, North Carolina. You were the first "outsiders" to critique *The Dog Diet* and affirm my belief in the project.

Mikki Voisard, fellow author and dog enthusiast. Your support and advice early on gave me hope and led me to my artist, your husband, David Voisard, who, though 3,000 miles away, captured the spirit of Sadie and our story in his wonderful illustrations.

A special thanks and my gratitude to the PetSmart Love-A-Pet Adoption program, without which I would never have found Sadie.

And last, but by no means least, my parents, Bill and Joanne Lawson. Your love, support and willingness to read all my writing over the years means everything.

INTRODUCTION

*B*ridget Jones had nothing on me. I got up and weighed myself in the middle of the night more times than I care to remember. I kept meticulous records of my meals and intake of calories, fat, protein, fiber and carbohydrates—except for the things I ate standing up, in the car or very late at night. Grapefruit diet, juice diet, egg diet, 4-Day Diet, no-carb diet, all-carb diet, no-meat diet, steak diet, cabbage soup diet, broth diet, tea diet, fasting . . . I tried them all. At any given time, along with a friend or two, I was trying out a new diet. I bought every diet supplement on the market as long as it had a "guaranteed or your money back" promise.

I'd spend hours in the grocery store filling my cart with endless combinations of foods that were going to do it for me "this time." After I'd reach the checkout, the process would start all over again, as I would grab and throw into my cart each and every magazine that even hinted of diet secrets that I was missing out on. Each time a new "miracle" was discovered, alas, the foods I had just stocked up on were not the right ones. "Okay," I'd say. "Eat these and just start this new strategy next week."

And on and on it went.

My obsession did not begin and end with food, however. I hired personal trainers, I ran, I walked, I stretched, I huffed and puffed, and I exhausted not only myself, but also everyone around me. I joined gyms and bought exercise equipment. I wore out a treadmill and kept an extra set of free weights in my car trunk for overnight stays. I joined contests and had before and after photos taken—or maybe I should say before and before photos. I once even tore a photo out of a family reunion scrapbook because I was too fat that year. I jumped on trampolines, ran up steps, stretched rubber bands, wrapped my thighs in plastic, suffered in steam rooms and walked across pools with ankle weights on. I had a collection of ab rollers, thigh masters and sauna suits.

I even associated major events in my life with whatever was or was not going into my mouth at the time. First wedding? Oh yes, I was on the champagne-only diet. (The champagne diet also served as a good excuse for that first-wedding fiasco.) Graduation from law school? Sure I look happy in the photo—not only had I just gotten my law degree, I had spent the last two weeks on cabbage soup and had entered that blissful euphoria I imagine people must experience just before starving to death. First divorce? The 4-Day Diet— almost longer than my marriage.

It's true that misery loves company. I pulled and dragged along anyone I could on these diet adventures. My friend Marty and I would go to a juice-fasting spa in Key West. We never experienced the joy of a cheeseburger in paradise; however, we can tell you all about happy hours with potato water and sneaking into the spa's kitchen late at night for a morsel of solid food in the form of a grapefruit section. There was my mother, who sent me a refrigerator magnet that said "Square Meals Make Round People" and

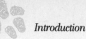

convinced me the key to dieting was in drinking apple cider vine-
gar first thing each morning. Bobi, my best friend, and I would
live on coffee for days, often because we had no money for anything else, but that is another story. Julie and I gorged on fat-free
foods; my sister and I lived for weeks on Alba 77 milkshakes.
Season and I experienced a nearly illegal high eating bacon, eggs,
"real" mayonnaise and cheeseburgers without buns.

And so it went until a little dog taught me some big lessons
about life. I met her one sunny Saturday when, during a crazy
period of my life, I cruised up to our local PetSmart in my pristine
Mercedes convertible. Now, understand, this is a car I have never
even let one person drink a clear liquid in, yet in a matter of less
than an hour I found myself tooling back down the highway with
a dog kennel on the backseat. In that kennel was a little black and
tan dog that I had promised to take care of for "one night."

I eventually named her Sadie, and she not only became my best
friend, she ended my crazy quest for the ultimate diet secret. With
Sadie I lost the weight I had lost over and over again for many years
. . . and this time I lost it for good. With Sadie I let go of the obsession for perfection and started enjoying my life in the most unexpected ways. Sadie pulled me from a bleak depression, lightened up
my mind and my body as well.

So, if you are like I was, you're probably wondering, "But what
did you *do*? What should I *eat*?" While this book will have some
food suggestions, it goes way beyond these. You will see how to rev
up your metabolism and slow down your life. I will show you how
Sadie taught me to find joy in simple things, and in doing so, I

found out that I was not a number on a scale, a perfectly balanced meal or a five-mile run. I hope my experience of saving a small dog, who in turn saved me, will inspire you, encourage you and most of all make you laugh—at yourself!

PART ONE

Shedding Pounds

CHAPTER ONE

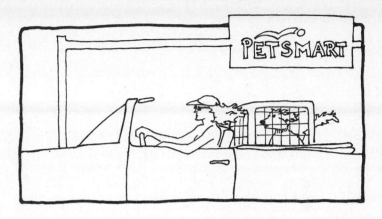

Misery Seeks Company

(And I thought things couldn't get worse)

$\mathcal{F}$orget what Charles Dickens said, "It was the best of times, it was the worst of times." The winter of 2002 was just plain the *worst of times*. I was fresh off a broken romance. It was the coldest winter the East Coast had seen for years. The country was on the brink of war, and I was on my couch, miserable, wallowing in self-pity. There was no measure to the depth of my dejection. My bleak days began and ended with tears. I read travel magazines, longing to go somewhere warm, but knowing my body was nowhere near bathing-suit ready. To improve this, I made halfhearted attempts to get motivated by trying various new weight-loss strategies, but I fell terribly short of implementing anything long enough to see even the merest result.

Instead, I comforted myself with mashed potatoes, a most excellent cold-weather comfort food; Starbucks ice cream, which really doesn't make you cold if you eat it wrapped up in a blanket in front of the fireplace; and, of course, the ultimate food for melancholy, chocolate. I had chocolate in every room of my house, in every form imaginable. Hershey's Kisses, Godiva Seashells filled with chocolate cream, Hershey's Almond Bars, raspberry-filled chocolate bars, white chocolate mints from a favorite candy store back home and, of course, chocolate peanut butter cups. I even had chocolate coffee and a chocolate-scented bubble bath. When everything got to be too much, I just stocked up on more chocolate.

I spent hours reading depressing literature and memorized pertinent passages to provide validation for my dejected condition. I wallowed in my misery, much like Matthew Arnold described in the last lines of his poem "Dover Beach," where he saw "neither joy, nor love, nor light, nor certitude, nor peace, nor help for pain." I was absolutely inconsolable.

My home had become an unbearably lonely prison. I sat in my pristinely clean palace jail, longing for any form of living company and started thinking that maybe the idea of getting a dog had some merit. If I was going to be miserable, I no longer wanted to do it alone. Even a dog might be better than this solitary isolation.

As many people who know me well will tell you, I was absolutely the last person on earth anyone would even think should ever have a dog. For the first four years that I owned my house, no one was allowed in with their shoes on. I called repair men to fix only things located in the basement because it had an exterior door. I didn't want them tracking into my house with dirty shoes and tools. I even sat on the floor in front of my new sofa for over a year—it was light colored, and I didn't want to get it dirty. I always hung up my clothes, washed the dishes immediately after using them, and my linen closet looked like it belonged to Martha Stewart.

My yard was also meticulously groomed. When I bought the house, I inherited a yard guy named Roy. I gave him detailed instructions about picking up grass clippings, keeping leaves off the lawn, weeding the roses and watching for trespassing dogs. I detested the thought of a dog trampling my flowers, or worse, taking a bathroom break in the front yard.

As a professional single woman, I loved to travel, and I enjoyed, or so I thought, having no one to consider when planning a getaway. I often bragged that I liked the fact that when I went home and turned the key in the lock, there were no surprises and no one there to disturb me. I ate when I felt like it (which took up a lot of my time), went to the gym unencumbered, stayed out as long as I wanted.

Ah, and then that winter of my discontent found me unsettled, wasting away in my near-sterile environment. This perfect setting no longer held solace or joy for me. I was the lone prisoner of my own entrapment.

Spring found me pudgy and pitiful, feeling my life was worthless and without promise. It was in the midst of this disjointed condition that I, neatness-obsessed, control-freak, type A personality, did something totally out of character. I got a dog.

And so, I emerged that rare, sunny Saturday in March. The sun had reappeared after a very long absence, and I was tooling along in my recently detailed convertible to PetSmart. Yes, the crazy idea that a dog might lift me out of my doldrums somehow had been occupying my idle thoughts. I was just going to get a look. After all, to be out of the gray fleece robe I had lived in all winter and not lying on the couch with a cup of hot chocolate was a step in the right direction.

Once in PetSmart, the din of dogs and kids should've been enough to cause my hasty retreat, but I didn't leave. Cautiously, I made my way over to the area where the local animal shelter brought homeless cats and dogs in for adoption. I observed from a distance as kids hovered around the fence with the puppies, and a volunteer walked an older dog around meeting prospective "parents." One of the volunteers was busy talking to a few people while holding some sort of puppy over her shoulder. I thought I would get a closer look at what was behind the fence where the children hovered when it happened.

"Here," the volunteer said as I passed, "just hold her for a minute while I help these people." I looked around thinking she must be talking to someone behind me. She was not, and suddenly I was holding this little dog at arm's length, much the way I'd held the baby or two that had been thrust upon me in the past. I thought if I didn't look at this dog, the "minute" would soon be over, and I could hand her back. But the "minute" did not end, and I looked at her . . . this little black and tan creature eyeing me warily.

Two dark brown eyes stared at me from beneath tan eyebrows with wild black hairs that reminded me of spider legs. Her eyes had a suspicious expression—you know, like your high school teacher used to give you when she was trying to decide if you had broken a rule. She had floppy ears covered with hair resembling a bad permanent wave. But it was her little licorice black nose that quivered ever so slightly, discerning my perfume, that got to me. Something about that dainty nose was quite endearing, and I relaxed my arms and drew her closer to me. She was softer than any cashmere sweater I had ever worn. I held her over my shoulder, braced for the inevitable tongue licking I detested from dogs, but it didn't come. Warily, she put both paws on my shoulder and pushed herself back to look into my face—what was this little dog doing? She just kept her paws on my shoulder, keeping a distance between us, and she studied me.

I felt the sharpness of her toenails digging through my sweater, which I realized was probably getting snagged beyond repair, but I couldn't move. I could feel her little breaths on my face, and I tried to figure out what she was thinking. Better yet, what was I thinking?

The last thing I needed, I realized, was a dog, albeit a cute one with a surprisingly intelligent manner. When my romance had ended the previous fall, my world became a maze of misplaced dreams. Nothing seemed to make sense anymore or fit into any of the many rigid patterns that made up my life. I couldn't see any of my numerous accomplishments, just discarded diets, procrastination and failures. I dragged myself to work, overwhelmed with the many responsibilities of my job. I simply had no spare time to care for a dog when I was doing such a poor job of caring for myself. I spent my time feeling sorry for myself and worrying about the future.

The pet shelter volunteer came back after what seemed the longest minute in the world and started putting things away. She suddenly remembered me and said, in a breezy manner, "Oh, well, do you want her?" Want her, I gasped silently, I don't even know really *what* she is. I quickly composed myself and in my lawyer persona said that I really liked her (lawyers never lie you know), but it was impossible to make a decision of such magnitude so quickly, and thanks, but here she is. The volunteer just ignored my spiel and kept picking up papers and clearing off the table set up for the adoption transactions. "Well, we really don't like to send them back to the shelter on Saturday nights because they just have to come back here tomorrow, so why don't you take her home with you for the night?" I felt panic as I never had before, even on the night before a trial. However, instead of protesting, for reasons I haven't yet discovered, I asked what I had to do, and before I knew it, there she was in the backseat of my car.

I'd heard stories of how "grateful" shelter dogs were just to get a home and how some people felt this instant bond with the adopted animal. Such was not my case. This dog was quite reserved in her consideration of me for her "mom," as the shelter volunteer called

me, and with my house for her home. There was no
tail wagging, no wild joyous running around, no
immediate acceptance by her for me or me for her.

That first night she was, at best, cordial to me. I usually go to the refrigerator as soon as I am in the door of
my house. But now I had the little dog to care for. So I
fed her first. I gave her some of the food that had been
sent along with her from PetSmart. She sniffed it and then ignored
it. I got her some water in a Styrofoam cup, and as she drank it,
sounded like a drain unclogging when the Liquid-Plumr has finally
worked. I was amazed at how this dainty little dog could lap up
water with such gusto. I smiled watching as she ran around the
kitchen sniffing everything. I should've recognized that something
was happening here. It was Saturday night and instead of planning
a melancholy lonely feast, I was not hungry, and I was smiling.

I placed her small pet carrier in the kitchen and took her for a
walk. No leash or collar? No problem. I slipped one of my terry
headbands over her head and made a leash from a garden cord. I
was beginning to get this dog thing down rather quickly, I thought.

I live two short blocks from our state capitol. The neighborhood
is an eclectic mix of single-family homes, apartments and houses
that have been converted into offices for small government depart-
ments and lobbyists. My house, like the others in the area, is a large,
three-story brick colonial. Much too large for one person, I bought
it because it was a good deal and within walking distance to my job
as a government attorney at the State Capitol Complex. It is also
one block from the Kanawha River, where there is a jogging path,

and where people walk their dogs. After stress-filled workdays, I'd usually just dash out my front door, straight to the boulevard for a fast four-mile walk. Today though, there would be no dashing, because I had this small dog on the end of a garden cord.

So we strolled through the neighborhood on an uneventful, but interesting, walk. She looked everything over carefully. She stuck her head through the fence next door and examined the cat. She ran around the perimeters of the yards we passed. I noticed a neighbor already had a small plot prepared for a garden and a house was for sale. We walked down the boulevard and past the capitol, where she captured the attention of the capitol police. She jumped up into the yard at the governor's mansion. The splendor of the lovely Georgian colonial house was lost on her as she took a pee. I looked anxiously at the security camera's angle and hurried her on. Then I laughed. I admired her nonchalant attitude about peeing in the governor's yard. My small tour guide was showing me things I walked by every day and never saw.

Bedtime arrived soon enough, and I placed a soft towel in her crate, put her inside and shut the door. I went about my usual bedtime routines and got in bed only to hear unbelievable noises coming from the kitchen. At first I thought that my security system had somehow malfunctioned, sending these horrendous sounds in all directions. It was incomprehensible to me that this delicate little dog had turned into a howling, mad wolf in less than a half hour.

Down I went, turned on the kitchen light, opened the crate door and out she came and just sat there looking at me. *What does she want?* I asked myself. Turning to my own solution for troubled times, I opened the refrigerator. The contents were sparse, so I reached into the freezer and gave her an ice cube. I thought that maybe, just maybe, it would keep her busy. She immediately began crunching it up, so I gave her a second one and pushed her back into the crate, shut the door, turned off the light and went back upstairs to bed.

I didn't quite make it back into bed before that horrendous barking, howling and banging up against the crate door began all over again. What was going on here? How could these gigantic sounds be coming from a dog that weighed less than I'd ever tried to lose in one day?

I ran back down the stairs repeating the routine, and once again she just popped out the crate door, sat down and stared at me. *This is it,* I decided. *You're going to the basement.* I picked up the crate, put the dog under one arm and down we went. I placed the crate as far away from the laundry chute as I could, hoping the wailing would not carry up the tin-lined shaft to the second floor outside my bedroom. I told her it was time to go to sleep, turned on the television timer, left on a small light and went back upstairs, confident that this would be the end of it.

I was no sooner in bed when it all started up again. Howling, crying, barking—it was worse than a nightmare because I was awake. I opened the laundry chute door and looked down. No, she had not somehow gotten loose and was not standing under the shaft directing all her vocal power up to me . . . it just sounded louder as I listened through the megaphone effect. I realized *nothing* I did was going to silence this dog, so I tried instead to ignore it. After all, it was only for tonight. I slammed shut the laundry chute door, closed my bedroom door, downed three Tylenol PMs, put my own television on timer and, for good measure, turned on my sound machine to "thunderstorm." Then I shut off the lights and lay back down to attempt sleep.

In no time, I was jerked awake by howling even louder than it had been earlier. I was confused . . . was I dreaming . . . why would I be having a dream of howling dogs . . . was it morning? Then it hit me. Oh, yes, that dog from PetSmart was *still* here. I guess I was expected to take her out, but how could it be morning already? I looked at the clock. It was not. I could not believe it. It was 4:30 A.M.! Surely dogs don't have to pee in the middle of the night. But then again, what if they do? Or worse. I'd have to clean that crate. I certainly wasn't up for that.

I put on my old, gray fleece robe, ran down the stairs, put my fur coat on over it and proceeded to the basement. There sat the source of all my troubles. This little dog's sweet face and dainty size certainly belied what I knew now to be her true character. I opened her crate door and she ran out and up the stairs. As I stumbled up the stairs after her, she ran back, peeked down at me and barked.

What an ungrateful brat! Here I was in the middle of the night taking care of her, but I was obviously not doing it fast enough. I took her outside saying, "You better really have to pee, or I am going to be even madder than I am right now."

Luckily for her, she did have bathroom duties

to attend to, and as I shivered in the March night air, I could only think that when I'd thought things couldn't get worse, they had. Here I was outside on a dark, cold night with a strange dog. I couldn't believe I'd actually brought this on myself. The dog and I ran back into the house as I counted how many hours until the woman would be back at PetSmart, and this dog would be back with her, and I would be free to lie back down on the couch and forget all about improving my situation.

Before I could grab her and take her back down to the basement, she ran into the kitchen ahead of me and headed straight for her food bowl. At last I had something in common with her: I too ate in the middle of the night. While she was quickly finishing up her food, I reached in the fridge to help myself to the last slice of pizza. She immediately began jumping on me, and I ended up giving her my extra-cheese, mushroom-covered treasure, hoping it would help her sleep. I returned her to the basement, the howling commenced, but I simply dragged myself back to bed and, finally, somehow, to sleep.

I was once again jolted awake by her cries at 7:00 A.M. *It's Sunday,* I thought. *It's only 7:00 A.M. . . . and I'm up?* The five hours until the adoption center at PetSmart would open stretched endlessly before me. I envisioned myself and this dog making countless trips in and out and up and down the basement stairs. Oh well, I had only promised to take care of her for one night, and although it might have been the longest night of my life, it would soon come to an end. Dragging myself up, I thought I might as well just get the rest of the day going until I could return her.

I stumbled down to the basement to get her. She ran friskily out of the carrier, did a few laps around my feet, bit the hem of my fur coat (which I had evidently slept in after our nocturnal outing) and scampered up the stairs. *How could she be awake, let alone so cheerful?* I wondered groggily. I took her outside and returned to the kitchen to make some coffee. I examined the contents of the refrigerator. It held only milk and a Hershey bar that I could not—would not—share with her. Because my Saturday night had been consumed with this dog, I had not stocked my refrigerator with my usual gluttonous foods and had no leftovers from a take-out meal either. I gave her the milk, which she drank as loudly as she had the water the night before. Surely, she could wait a few hours until we returned to PetSmart where they would feed her.

I took my coffee and Sunday paper to the living room and proceeded to ignore her. I hoped she might fall asleep (at which point I could too), but no such luck. Following on my heels over to the sofa, where I set out my paper, she scurried up and began tugging at sections. Of course, only the sections I wanted to read. She grabbed the "Life and Style" section and ran around the couch with it. It was the section I always read first. I was particularly interested in it this day, as my first feature travel story was going to be in it. I grabbed the section from her, quickly turned the pages and there was my story in its entire splendor! I began reading, getting lost in my own memories of the time I'd spent at this lovely spa and was now sharing with what I imagined to be hundreds of thousands of readers. Even this dog couldn't dampen my elation at seeing my words in print.

After another walk, I put her in the crate and headed back to PetSmart. No way could I keep this dog. One night and I was in worse shape than I had been in the previous morning. No, someone else will make a much better "mom" for this creature. I was imagining the many travel stories I would write in the months to come. What would I do with a dog while traveling to these luxurious and exotic locales? Surely traveling and writing would snap me out of this miserable, heartbroken melancholy, and I wouldn't need a dog. She simply could not stay.

Inside the store, I located the woman who had foisted this dog off on me. In my most gracious manner, I explained how I just wasn't the right person for the dog, and that I felt bad keeping her any longer while she could be on display here. She was so cute, she'd undoubtedly get an absolutely great home and have an even greater life. Sorry, etcetera, etcetera. I'm gone.

I ran on the boulevard that Sunday. I ate a pound of jerked shrimp, a mushroom pizza and a pint of mocha java chip ice cream in front of the TV. I took a bubble bath. I went to bed early, but I couldn't sleep. I went into the hall and opened the laundry chute door. Silence. No TV. No barking.

I missed her. Darn. What was going on here? Where was she sleeping tonight? Was she back at the shelter? Was she auditioning another prospective "mom"? *She really was cute, wasn't she?* Maybe I didn't need so much sleep after all. And wasn't she just the softest little creature I had ever touched? I walked down the two flights of stairs to the basement and stood where her little crate had sat. My sense of loss was unreasonable. I was used to feeling lonely and sad these past many weeks, but this was different.

I went up to the kitchen to look in the refrigerator . . . one of my insomniac habits developed in the past winter months. The plate I'd used for her was still sitting on the floor. I picked it up and put it in the garbage. *Wasn't that just the funniest way she drank her water?* I slowly walked back upstairs. *It really was cute the way she ran up the basement stairs and then came back looking for me.*

Monday morning came, and I didn't want to get out of bed. There was nothing to look forward to; it was cold, the sun wasn't shining, and I was wondering what in my closet would fit me. I arrived at my office late, but hey, I was at least there. Sitting at my desk, I started thinking . . . *what kind of terrible person am I that I can't even make room for a little dog in my big house? I'd probably get to work on time if I had that dog, wouldn't I?* Okay, maybe the dog wasn't crazy about me either, but what was going to happen to her? Then again, what was going to happen to me? Things were bleak: No husband. Overweight. A job that had become boring. But, no, a dog would just add to this dilemma my life had turned into. I had been neglecting everything lately, how could I take care of her? I certainly wasn't the right "mom" for this dog.

"Putnam Animal Shelter," the friendly voice on the other end of the phone said. I explained my purpose for calling.

"You had one of our puppies, and you took her back?"

"Well, yes," I stammered. "I'd felt pressured to decide too quickly whether I wanted her. I mean, maybe I'm not the best home for her, and she barked most of the night, and I think she ate some of the newspaper I was reading, which worried me. I took her back . . . because . . . well . . . is she there? I think I do want her."

She wasn't. None of the puppies had come back from PetSmart, so she had probably been adopted. I was most welcome to come and pick another dog. "But, you never know," I heard her saying, "Give me your phone number in case something comes up."

See, I told myself. *Nothing is ever going to work out for you again. You have an endless life of cold winters ahead filled with unsuccessful diets, sometime boyfriends and a pension in about twenty years.* With those discouraging thoughts, I headed for the cafeteria. Two pancakes, two eggs and four slices of bacon later, I returned to my office. My secretary buzzed me and said, "Why is the Putnam Animal Shelter looking for you?"

It seems that the volunteer had a suspicion that I was the right "mom" for this little dog. She'd taken her home for the night anticipating that I would change my mind. Betty, the volunteer, said that if I wanted "Katie" (that was what she called the dog), I could meet her at Wendy's near her home with $40 and the dog would be mine. I shouted at the receptionist that I would be right back and ran home to get my car.

As I drove out to meet Betty that cold March day, the sun came out. I arrived first and spent several anxious minutes examining cars as they pulled in. Finally, I spotted a car with Betty behind the wheel, and the small, dark shape of a dog at the passenger window.

I handed over $40 and signed the adoption papers right there in the parking lot. I put her in the car and drove back to the office. I didn't know if dogs were allowed in my building or not, but I put her in my big tote bag and in we went.

Everyone in the office wanted to see her. I put her down on the floor and she proceeded to check everyone out and sniffed her new surroundings. I hurriedly finished a few tasks while she played with a roll of tape on the floor of my office.

I was soon headed back to PetSmart. But this time, we were going shopping. I started thinking that I should give her a new name. I couldn't call her Katie because one of my sisters once had a perfectly hateful mother-in-law named Katie, so the name Betty had given her carried some unfortunate associations. I didn't call her anything. I couldn't think of a name. We shopped and left the store loaded down with a new crate, puppy chow, assorted toys and chews, and a brand-new red leash and collar. Our demeanor toward each other was guarded at best. She seemed ticked off at me for callously returning her, and I was unsure if this adoption would work out.

As a person with no experience taking care of a dog, I did the best I could, and that simply didn't feel good enough. During those first few weeks together, I was constantly tired. I never knew if I fed her enough or fed her too much. She got stubborn and wouldn't eat at all. I coaxed her with treats. She howled every night and never wanted to go into her "pennie" as I called it. Anywhere between 3:00 and 4:30 A.M., I would jerk awake from the sounds of her sharp barking. Same routine every night—reach for glasses, put on

long, gray, fleece robe, stumble to first floor, put
on my fur coat, down to basement, open pennie . . .
back up basement stairs, out back door and through
yard gate to the designated pee place.

I almost forgot these nightly outings by the
time morning rolled around. In the light of day
they seemed almost surreal, until one 3:00 A.M. a capitol policeman
came by as I waited for her to pee. I knew all the officers; I encountered them daily going to and from work, and my house is adjacent
to a state-owned building and large parking lot.

"We've gotten quite a kick out of seeing you on these little
midnight runs. Watching you and your little dog has become our
favorite pastime. In fact, we think you look rather cute in this
getup," he said.

In complete humiliation, I realized that I'd forgotten about the
surveillance cameras that cover my house and the parking lot
twenty-four hours. I had forgotten the security room filled with
monitors that the officers watched diligently during their shift.
There in that room banked with televisions, I had become a star.

I wanted my life back. I called Betty. "I'm not sure this is working out. I don't think she likes me."

"What did you name her?" she wanted to know.

"Well, I haven't named her yet."

"Give her a name; it will get better." Betty's brief advice was
no help.

I went to the grocery store one day after work, forgetting that the
dog was at home, and I suddenly remembered that I needed to let

her out. I hurried through the store, forgetting half my stuff. I felt trapped. Yes, I wanted my life back.

I would make lunch plans and leave before eating, remembering the dog was at home still in her pen. I asked a friend to watch her so I could go for a *real* walk/run, because she was too little to go four miles. When I returned, he was frantic. She had scratched at the door the entire time I was gone. If I wanted to take a bubble bath, her cries would echo up from the basement through the laundry chute, negating any soothing effect the chocolate milk bath might have delivered.

I wanted to go to bed early, but she would want to go outside. I wanted to talk on the phone; she seemed to hate the phone and would bark incessantly. When I'd go to mail my bills at the post office, I'd leave her in the car. I was embarrassed by her barking as I'd leave her to go into the building. It wasn't as if the dog was in ecstasy when she was in my presence. Quite the opposite. For the most part she ignored me, yet she didn't want me out of her sight. This was beginning to have some familiar aspects of my dating life.

I now knew with certainty, beyond all questions, why I'd never had a child and why couples who have babies to save their marriages usually split up. It was overwhelming, all consuming, and even my depressed, vegetative winter hibernation seemed a more desirable condition. I was still stumbling through my life; but now I had company . . . company that required constant attention, which was very small consolation.

Betty called me at my office. Ah, I thought, could all my frustration be over? Is it possible that her previous parent had changed her mind about giving her up?

"How's Katie doing?" she asked.

"Well, I don't call her Katie."

"What have you named her?"

"Nothing. I just don't think this is working out, and if she has to get used to a new home, she should have the new 'mom' give her a name."

Then I noticed a change in her voice. "I'm not calling to see if she's working out. I need to know how she is. Is she sick?"

Sick? I thought. "No, I don't think so." With all her energy and bright spirit, this dog was actually the picture of health.

"She might have a few psychological problems. I mean she wakes me up every night, I can't even eat around her, and she doesn't want to be out of my sight, and when I take her in the car . . ."

"No, Patti. I need some serious answers here. Is she sick? Does she have a fever? Is she eating? Does she have diarrhea? Is she lethargic?"

"No, no, yes, no, no," I answered.

"Well, are you sure?" she continued.

"As far as I know, but you know I'm no dog expert."

I mean, after all, I was a dog illiterate. I suddenly realized I didn't know enough about dogs to have one.

"You know," I said, "you should have asked me some things about myself. I was pretty depressed this winter, and it would've probably been better for me to have waited to get this dog. I mean, I doubt any psychiatrist would certify me dog-parent material." I hate to admit it, but at this point I would have latched onto any reason for returning the dog.

And then I listened . . . it was unbelievable. Betty told me that all the other puppies that had been at PetSmart with this little dog had died. *Died? Puppies die? How?* This dog was so full of life; she was a perpetual fur ball of energy, to be more exact.

"They all got parvo," she continued. Something, of course, that I knew nothing about. Betty explained that parvovirus was a fatal dog disease. Because this dog had not gone back to the shelter the night I kept her, she may have been spared. Betty cautioned me to keep an eye on the dog, and if she developed any symptoms, to get her to the vet at PetSmart right away.

Suddenly, all the images of this dog that had been swallowed up in feedings, bathroom trips, early risings, barking and begging came dancing before my eyes. Her joyful spirit each morning. Her cautious regarding of me, almost sensing that this tenuous arrangement between us might not be permanent.

The delicate way she took her treats and the equally quick snap of her mouth when she crunched an ice cube. How she stood on her hind legs and twirled around in the kitchen, happy to see her breakfast. How she gobbled her food so quickly and then wanted mine. How she never missed the smell of anything remotely signifying food or came running at the sound of the refrigerator. The way she still dashed up the basement steps and then ran back to peek down to see if I was coming too. The little teeth marks on my tulips and the chew toys scattered around the house. The place mat on the kitchen floor that her little, shiny stainless steel food and water bowls sat on and her leash hanging on the baker's rack. The towel on the back porch to dry her paws off with, and the way she looked when she was wet from her bath.

It was all dear to me. I was no longer greeted by silence when I opened the door to my formerly clinically clean house, which was now disheveled. My house had gone from clean to comfortable, and I had hardly noticed. Her possessions and mine alike were scattered around in domestic familiarity. I now had a home . . . and so did she.

I left the office and ran all the way home in my high heels. I realized this little dog needed me. She depended on me. It mattered to her if I slept in or chose to lie on the couch all day. And it became so clear to me that I needed her, and I loved her.

I opened the front door, shut off the alarm and yelled, "MOM IS HOME" as I ran down the basement steps. There she was, clinging to the side of her little pennie, barking and wriggling wildly. I opened the door and instead of pushing her down, I caught her as she jumped up, and as I hugged her, I realized how very precious she had become to me.

I quickly gathered her leash and my purse, and we got into the car and headed for PetSmart. I wanted the veterinarian to check her out. I couldn't wait around to see if she got sick. I wanted to know now that she was going to be okay.

The checkup was performed with the vet and his assistant saying what a good dog she was and how cute she was, and I was suddenly proud that she was my dog. I bought her a bag of chews, an extra box of treats and some disinfectant wipes for her paws. For good measure, I picked out some piña colada–scented shampoo and perfume, and we went home, together, in more ways than one.

Returning home, I didn't go to the basement and put her in the crate; instead I carried her up to my bedroom, so I could change clothes. Passing the spare bathroom, I noticed my three scales. Yes, *three*. A digital one, a standard scale and a high-tech one that also measures body fat. I realized I couldn't remember the last time I'd been on any of them. I'd been weighing myself at least once a day for most of my adult life, and now I didn't know how much I weighed.

Now, anyone who is constantly struggling with weight will tell you that you *never* weigh yourself in the afternoon. First thing in the morning is the lightest you will be all day, and that's the time to see what the numbers are. I realized it must have been over three weeks since I'd weighed myself—the length of time I had the dog. (Time flies even when you are *not* having fun.) Unthinkable. My morning routine was set in stone. Get up, pee and get on the scale. Drink coffee, run on treadmill or outside, weigh in again, just in case I'd either misread the scale numbers or burned off enough calories to register half a pound lighter. I'd followed this routine daily for more years than I could count, and here I was, realizing I hadn't followed it for almost a month.

So, I went for it. I thought that the afternoon sun was distorting the numbers on the first scale, so I got on the high-tech one. No. It was the same. Well, not really, because I knew the difference between the three scales; they never said the same thing, but I had this all mentally calibrated. Then I got on the old standard. What was going on here? I ran to the mirror. According to all three scales, I had lost eight pounds. How had *that* happened?

I ran into my home office and picked up the daily food journal where I recorded what I ate, the number of calories, fat, carbs, protein and fiber. Each page was a meticulous record of that day's activities, weight and positive or negative calorie intake. I also recorded other things that could influence my weight. For example, if I had gotten stressed out and eaten a container of ice cream, drank a whole bottle of wine or made three trips to the Indian buffet at lunch. But the pages had not been written on for the past few weeks. I couldn't figure out what was going on. Had I been in a coma? Was I presently in a dream?

I got out a pair of jeans that I'd thought I'd never be able to wear again. At my worst, I couldn't get them over my hips, and at my best had to zip them up with a fork. This time, although by no means did they slip on easily, I was able to pull them up, and I could zip them without using a fork. Okay, so maybe I couldn't sit down in them, but hey, this was still major progress.

It couldn't be a dream, could it, if these jeans were here and I had them on? How had this happened? I started thinking back over the last three weeks and there the dog sat looking at me. I couldn't sit down (I still had the jeans on), so I stood and looked at her. Had this dog had anything to do with this? I started wondering.

I thought of the horrible winter, and it dawned on me that I didn't feel so bad anymore. In fact, since I'd become consumed with caring for this dog, I couldn't remember not wanting to get out of bed in the morning or gorging on chocolate.

I struggled out of the jeans and changed my clothes while still trying to figure out what had happened to me. Everything had seemed so terrible, and everything had been such a blur until today. Maybe

I'd never figure it out, but for better or worse, I had this little dog, and not only did I feel better, I was eight pounds lighter. We were in this together; I just had no idea what exactly we were in. I was about to learn some big lessons about life and dieting and myself from this little, nameless dog that had turned my life inside out.

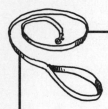

Dog Diet
DISCOVERIES

1. Dogs make some things harder, but everything better.

2. Dogs give unexpected, unrequested, unconditional love.

3. Dogs get you off the scale and onto the sidewalk!

4. A house becomes a home when it goes from clean to comfortable.

5. Dogs make you unaware that you are even dieting!

CHAPTER TWO

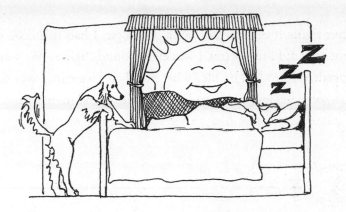

The Bark Alarm

(Rejoicing in the morning)

I was so grateful to this little dog for my eight-pound weight loss. My mission was to discover exactly what role she had played in making these pounds evaporate. By examining what we had been doing together, I'd reveal the secret and continue to become the skinny me I had longed to recapture for years. In the process, we'd become like Lassie and Timmy—great friends, forever. However, our bonding was not so easily accomplished.

The morning after the parvo scare, her shrill barks filtered up through the laundry chute. Her pennie was still in the basement where, I hoped, her barking would eventually become so faint that I wouldn't be able to hear it in my second-floor bedroom. Each night I was optimistic as I handed her a bribe in the form of a Milk-Bone, locked her in the crate, put her television on timer—Animal Planet of course—and trudged up to the second floor to begin my own bedtime ritual. I had stuffed the laundry chute with old pillows in a feeble attempt to muffle her endless barking. She weighed only eight pounds at this time, the exact amount of weight I had lost, and I still marvel at how she could produce such a high volume with her barks. I felt like someone who had just been handed a life sentence and sees "This is the first day of the rest of your life" scrawled on the prison cell wall.

I've never been a morning person, and all I wanted was to sleep in just a little bit longer. The previous evening had been a joyous celebration of her good health and my jeans fitting. But now, in the cold light of day, I had to get up because she wanted to go out. Her barking grew louder, and I hauled myself up to see what was so urgent.

It was at times like these, when things seemed unbearable between us, that I'd hold her in front of the mirror imagining the eight pounds back on my body. It made me grateful, and having a lively, wriggling, eight-pound example to show myself exactly what I'd accomplished was great.

I realized I needed to give her a name. I made a list of all the dog names I'd heard before, but none of them seemed right. At her vet's office, her records still said "New Puppy." Each time we went for one more of what seemed like endless puppy vaccines, they gave me curious looks and could not understand why I had yet to produce a name for this dog who was a favorite at the clinic.

She was so cute that she garnered lots of attention on our walks, and everyone's first question was, "What's her name?" My answer that I hadn't given her one yet was fine for the first few weeks, but grew embarrassing after that.

Rodney, my neighbor/ex-boyfriend (those of you who have had the misfortune to experience this combination will appreciate my dilemma here), had several suggestions that were impossible. He thought she was a jubilant little dog, which she was, and wanted me to call her Jubil. I couldn't do it. It didn't fit. He started calling her all sorts of stupid names, and she'd respond to any of them.

It was in these early weeks that I had to leave the dog with Rodney for several days. I'd reserved and paid for my annual after-tax-return trip to Hilton Head Island long before the dog came into my life. In the past, whether a property allowed dogs or not had never been a factor. But, like everything else in my life, this was now different. Dogs were strictly forbidden where I was going, and unless I wanted to be at the mercy of my ex-husband who lives on the island and leave the dog at his house, I couldn't take her with me.

So, promises of many dinners and breakfasts got Rodney to agree to care for her while I went off to the beach. I was so relieved and, more than anything else, looking forward to finally sleeping in. During my week at Hilton Head, I slept uninterrupted. The lovely sound of the ocean replaced the dog's morning barking. It was heavenly. I felt a few pangs of guilt for abandoning her so soon during our residency together, so as I was leaving the island, I stopped in at a pet store. I returned to Charleston rested, loaded down with dog gifts and surprised by the joyful reunion we had.

I certainly wasn't prepared to hear from a neighbor, "Hey, you finally gave her a name, but how on earth did you ever come up with the name Buckwheat?"

I wasn't one bit amused to learn that in my absence, Rodney had decided to try not one, but two names out on the dog. Buckwheat was bad enough, but the other name was Booger. I might not have been able to select a name, but his were outrageous. To make matters worse, she was starting to answer to either one of these ridiculous names. I was also afraid that she'd soon think her name was "Shut Up"—that's what I yelled down the laundry chute every morning as I tried to get a measly fifteen minutes more of sleep.

I couldn't believe that Rodney had taken it upon himself to get involved in the naming crisis in the first place. The day I brought her home from PetSmart, Rodney was the first person I showed her to. In my panic at actually having the dog in my possession, and overwhelmed with the thought of being responsible for another living creature, I had offered to make her a "joint dog."

We could share her—and the care of her. He had politely refused, saying that he couldn't handle the care of a dog, but thought she was cute and she would probably be good for me.

Why was I not surprised by this attitude? Rodney and I had dated for ten years. He'd also had other long-term girlfriends, but none of them, nor our relationship, had resulted in marriage. We tossed the idea around many times over the years, but neither one of us seemed to have the same thoughts at the same times, so, while the romance slowly fizzled out, we remained friends.

I was surprised, however, at how often he was now coming over to see "the dog." He played with her, took her riding in his convertible, got her all excited before bedtime and then went home. I had to do all the work. Once, when we had dropped by to visit him, she ran into the bedroom and peed on his bed before I could stop her. You would've thought she demolished the entire dwelling to hear him rant on about it. I had to haul the comforter across the street to my house to wash it immediately. There I was, with an unnamed dog pulling me along with her leash, while I struggled to hold on to a king-size comforter as we made our way through the parking lot and across the street. Maybe she did deserve one of those horrible names.

But, in the end, it was Rodney who finally came up with her name. Out of the blue, after I had considered more names than first-time parents most likely ever do, he casually said to me, "My grandmother's name was Sadie. She was so sweet and had such a kind disposition and lively spirit, and her name really fits this dog."

Sadie, I thought, as I looked at her sitting there looking at me. I tried it out. She jumped up on me, which, of course, meant nothing because she seemed to answer to anything by this time, but in that instant she became Sadie. It simply fit. The name brought on an avalanche of cute little nicknames, both endearing . . . and otherwise. She seemed very pleased that she was finally being called just one name, and in her own way rejoiced. I called her vet's office and told them. They approved.

Now that she was named, it was time to settle down and figure out this diet mystery with her. The fact that she now had a name, though, had no bearing on her continued early risings. Instead of yelling "shut up," I'd yell her name. Same effect—just more barking. The situation was getting critical. She always wanted out of the crate at an ungodly early morning hour. I was suffering the new-parent nightmare of sleep deprivation, and I didn't even have any doting grandparents to pawn her off on so I could sleep in just one morning. I longed to be back at the beach. My Sharper Image sound machine's weak faux ocean waves were no match for Sadie two floors below me.

This new obsession with sleep—or lack thereof—made me think back to one of my stretches of fitness fanaticism, when I had learned that to lose weight you needed to get eight hours of sleep. Although I never really grasped the technicalities of this phenomenon, it sounded good to me. To my dismay, the program didn't mean that you could sleep in. The personal trainer I was working with at the time insisted I meet her at the gym at 6:00 A.M. I spent twelve weeks shivering in the predawn West Virginia mornings that winter in hopes of a better body. It worked for a while, but like all my other efforts, it didn't last. My finances and my discipline both seemed to run out at the same time.

A different personal trainer, Dave, devised a regimen for me that unintentionally required a very early-to-bed plan. His rules didn't allow any eating after 7:00 P.M. That meant in order to obey his mandate I had to go to bed about 8:00 P.M., to avoid the inevitability of my eating something. I bargained at length with Dave about this, but, he assured me, this was essential in order to reach my goals. I never was able to completely abide by it. I simply could not go to bed early—or hungry.

Now with Sadie as my roommate, it was worse than living with either of these past fitness tyrants whom I'd paid dearly to shed a small amount of weight, and in a few short months I literally had nothing to show for my efforts. Sadie was forcing me to stay up late (bathroom duties), go to bed hungry (it was just too difficult to eat in peace around her) *and* get up early (more bathroom duties). I didn't see this arrangement lasting any longer than either of the trainers had. The only benefit was that Sadie didn't charge me by the hour.

But wait a minute; I felt enlightenment. *My new sleeping pattern* was part of the process that caused me to lose the eight pounds. I was employing the techniques of trainers that had gotten me into the best shape of my life, but I was doing it unconsciously. Sadie had succeeded where the trainers had failed; she made early morning exercise a part of my life. Looking through some materials I had from my training sessions, I was happy to discover actual validation for this morning exercise and weight loss result. I read that a study from Kansas State University had supposedly discovered that two-thirds of the calories you burn in the morning are from stored fat. Calories used up later in the day are only burning 50 percent from fat. Every little bit helps, and this small affirmation (true or not) was enough to keep me going.

Armed with my new information (which I'd chosen to believe), I began to approach this dog ownership deal differently. I was getting a free personal trainer in exchange for taking care of Sadie, which in retrospect maybe wasn't so bad after all. During those initial weeks when Sadie and I seemed to instinctively keep our distance from each other, housebreaking, feeding and keeping her quiet were all-consuming, but like getting up and walking early in the morning, these things were now part of my normal day's activities. At first, all these chores seemed to diminish the sudden rush of emotion that I'd felt the day I dashed off to the vet at PetSmart.

Most mornings, I was half-asleep when I got her out of her crate and took her outside. Once back inside, we'd both go on with our individual morning rituals. I'd return her to the basement crate and get ready for work. I came home at noon to walk her, and then we'd spend the evening going our separate ways. I'd work, read or watch television; she'd amuse herself with her growing inventory of toys.

Now a new routine developed with the morning risings. I had a purpose—I was losing weight. Sadie's first barks of the morning were a challenge to leap out of bed and begin the calorie-burning process. Our morning forays evolved into purposeful exercise walks, with Sadie at the end of her red leash calling the shots.

She never just ambled along. She frolicked, staring straight into the morning sun as she dragged me along with her. I was the holder of the leash, protecting her from the outside world of cars, bigger dogs and cats. She was the drill sergeant of the early-morning hours. She'd stand on her little hind legs at the sight of any person or thing that seemed interesting. Laughter began to replace my irritation at the early risings. These walks brought us both back to the house out of breath and ready for the day.

Once we returned to the house she always ran straight to her water dish and drained it with zest. I'd return her to her crate in the basement and then go upstairs to get ready for work. It wasn't that I didn't want to be closer to her. We had our moments of playing ball and lying on the couch together, but I was holding back. I didn't admit it to anyone, but despite her cheerful and genial attitude, I was a bit cautious, if not scared of her, in close quarters. This fear stemmed from a harrowing childhood experience when a neighbor's German shepherd attacked me.

I had dreams of the dog-biting incident for the longest time, and now here I was years later, with a black dog barking me awake every morning. I knew I needed to shake this last, lingering uncertainty I felt about her. Sadie couldn't know the history behind my reticent fear of her, and I, of course, despite joyful greetings and happy playtimes, didn't know what she thought of me. So we spent our time at arm's length from each other as we appraised our new living arrangement. I know at that time, even with her perhaps less than wonderful memories from the animal shelter, I was not the ideal dog mom she had perhaps dreamed about as she watched prospective parents parade by her cage. But my skills improved as my love for her grew, and had she given up that endless, annoying barking, we might not have taken so long to accept each other, but I simply could not stand the continual barking.

It was bad enough to fall asleep at night to this endless din, but in the morning, there was no escape. Her barking would well up through the laundry chute (the pillows didn't seem to muffle the sound one bit), making my mornings miserable. Barking over *The Today Show,* barking over the music I liked to play as I dressed, loudly barking over any phone conversations I attempted to have.

But one dreary, sleep-deprived morning, things finally changed. She howled. I got up. She tumbled out of her crate. All in the usual manner. Off we went on our morning excursion, but unlike all our previous days together, when we returned to the house, I took both Sadie and my coffee to my room with me to get ready for work. I was actually able to hear the television while she quietly played with her blue tennis ball. I was enjoying the sound of the shower water without any thought of barking or worry when something made me jump. Her blue tennis ball came rolling into the shower followed by her little head. She hated going out in the rain and quickly backed out of the shower with a puzzled expression. I swallowed some water from laughing under the spray, but I didn't care. I realized all she wanted was to be with me. Her presence in the bedroom as I got ready for work was comforting. In the end, we were two of a kind: someone had not wanted me, and someone had not wanted her, but here we were together, and things were going to be okay.

Mornings were finally under control, so I decided to try the same approach at night. I decided to let her sleep with me. Instead of taking her to her pennie at bedtime, I let her come upstairs with me. I put a sheet over the comforter, and then signaled to her that she was allowed up onto the bed. Up she hopped and made herself comfortable on the corner of the bed. I turned the TV on timer, climbed under the covers, and we fell asleep. Amusingly, I discovered that Sadie snored, but it was very brief and soft, nothing compared to the barking.

The next morning, I was not barked awake for the first time in what seemed like forever. She was just lying there looking at me when I woke up. We jumped out of bed together and a tug-of-war ensued when she kept taking my socks. I figured, what the heck, surely I must be burning more calories this way than simply putting on my socks. As a matter of fact, I realized that all of the extra activity with Sadie was another factor in my continued weight loss. These little workouts could just be another part of my fitness regimen with her.

By this time, Sadie weighed eleven pounds, and I had lost ten. I was surprised that she didn't weigh more because she was eating everything, and I was eating almost nothing. If this kept up, and I continued to lose the same amount of weight that Sadie was gaining, I was headed for slim city at last.

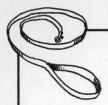

Dog Diet
DISCOVERIES

1. The sooner you get out of bed, the sooner you start burning calories.

2. Calories burned in the morning are more efficient at burning fat than those burned later in the day.

3. Laughing at your dog's antics is a great way to start your day.

4. If you want to get a good night's sleep, let your dog sleep with you.

5. Every morning is either the first or last morning of the rest of your life. It can be anything you make it.

CHAPTER THREE

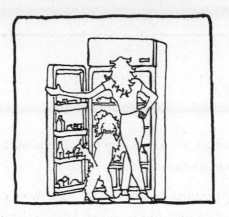

It's All About Eating

(First one on the floor gets the french fry)

Mornings were no longer just to be endured. They had a purpose in my renewed diet endeavors. Getting up early seemed to have a significant role in my initial weight loss, and I was enthused enough to continue the morning walks, with Sadie urging if not pulling me on. But there are two parts to most diet programs and exercise is only part of it. Food, or in my past experiences, the combinations and deprivations of it, was always the other part.

I had been a skinny kid. As a teenager I was flat-chested and downright scrawny. Then I turned thirty and everything changed.

No longer could I gorge on pizza, hot roast beef sandwiches, french fries and gravy, and hoagies. We had a restaurant in my hometown that made the best hoagies. The buns were hard on the outside, soft on the inside and always warm. Those sandwiches were so good my best friend once took two dollars out of her savings account just to buy them for our lunch. This place used only Hellmann's "real" mayonnaise, the brand I loved from my childhood. By the time I tried a popular low-carb program, I was convinced real mayonnaise was an illegal substance, but back then I enjoyed it. I had it on everything.

My honeymoon photos from my second wedding (the first marriage didn't last long enough for a honeymoon) show a still-thin girl in a cute red bikini frolicking in a private pool in Acapulco. It was shortly after this that the really obsessive dieting began. My husband and I operated a restaurant in Center City, Philadelphia. The food in our restaurant was delicious, and as the proprietor, every morsel in the place was available to me. Add to this that the entire second floor of the building was a gourmet food court, and those wonderful South Philly eateries with the famous cheesesteaks and Italian ices were just down the street. Tack on our forty-foot mahogany bar with the greatest downtown happy hour and free hors d'oeuvres, and I was in hog heaven. In short, I ate and I ate, and it caught up with me.

Every woman remembers that "first time," and I'm not talking about anything involving the opposite sex here. You know, the first time that favorite pair of worn-to-perfection jeans feels too tight. The jeans that feel like a warm blanket on a windy evening and have been everywhere with you. The ones you've thrown on the floor at night and hopped into again the next morning, and they always felt just right. Remember when Oprah finished her amazing weight loss from some sort of fasting scheme? What did she appear on national television wearing? HER JEANS! We monitor how we're doing in every aspect by how our jeans fit us.

It's a startling unfamiliar feeling when you step into your jeans and they aren't slipping on like your old shoes. This feeling quickly turns to sheer panic. You tug, then pull, and a few squirms later they're on and even zipped, but with difficulty. You immediately convince yourself that you washed them in hot water and dried them too long; that's what's wrong. A few hours of suffering in what feels like a straitjacket for the bottom half of your body, and the jeans feel a little more normal. Certainly that's what happened. It was the laundry.

Then it happens again, and the tug, squirm, pull routine once again brings the jeans to your waist with huge effort, but this time they won't zip. That's when you discover that forks have an unexpected useful purpose outside of the kitchen. The tine of the fork is perfect for gripping the zipper tongue, and if you lie back flat on your bed while keeping your feet on the floor, the jeans zip. And so it begins. The fork takes up permanent residence in your nightstand drawer; you begin zipping the jeans with the fork as a routine. Then one day the zipper breaks.

Yep, time to move up a size, and although you must purchase a larger size of jeans to appear in public, you hate it. How can this be? You've done nothing differently, but you are bigger! Of course, you keep the jeans because you're positive that you'll be able to wear them again. This is just a temporary condition. The excuses have become second nature at this point, but it's time for action whether you like it or not. Enter the world of dieting—and what a world it is.

One of my first diets was the 4-Day Diet. It sounded quite reasonable because I was *positive* my inflated condition was only a short-term situation, and in four days I could be on my merry way back into the size 4 jeans, and all those hoagies and pizzas would be forgiven. Although the food was distasteful, I reasoned, I could do anything for four short days, get into my dress for Saturday night, and I'd be done with it. So for four days, I had the restaurant chef prepare green beans, hard-boiled eggs and cauliflower for me. I would wash this down with grapefruit or prune juice. Of course I wouldn't eat these meals out in the restaurant, but in the tiny manager's office behind the kitchen, and for good measure I'd lock the door. Among the greasy recipes and invoices I'd forge through these bland meals. My suffering was a form of penance for my gluttony. Thus began the vicious cycle of all the crazy food combinations, fasting, coffee binges and worse, which lasted until the "winter of my discontent."

At one time or another I embarked on every extreme diet you can think of. You know, the one that promises you can eat whatever you want, never exercise and still lose weight in your sleep. Turns out the only people who ever lose weight in their sleep are in comas. Then there was the forty-eight-hour juice diet. You're provided with a small bottle of concentrated juice that you dilute with water and drink for forty-eight hours. That, too, proved ridiculous. I never heard of anyone who could even stand the taste of the juice, and any weight lost was merely from dehydration.

I was always on some sort of diet, restricted eating plan or new fitness regimen. I was ridiculous. I would deprive myself of the most basic enjoyments, only to break out and gorge on pizza until I was literally sick of it and sick of me.

When Sadie entered my life that winter nothing was off-limits to me where food was concerned. During that period, I had no intention of going on a diet. I'd let go of almost all food guidelines that had composed my eating life. My despair was so overwhelming I couldn't think of any future event that I needed to be in shape for. I was done with men and, therefore, felt I could also be done with dieting. I had no plans for dating someone new, no trips to a beach in the near future and, in general, my miserable mood just went better with a miserable body. I wasn't even inspired to slim down to fit into any of the numerous outfits hanging in my closet with the tags still on. You know—the ones we all have that we buy because they're on sale, but mainly because they are the size we want to be. But at that time the consequence of gaining weight didn't seem as important as comforting myself with every calorie-laden food that even looked like it might make me feel better.

Nor was exercise on my schedule that dismal winter. I wasn't even interested in walking. Charleston was having the coldest winter in years, so walking outside was not an option. I did manage to purchase a new treadmill, but the days my feet hit the belt were rare.

I soothed my shattered emotions with takeout from my favorite restaurants. I devoured shrimp from the Tidewater, gourmet pizzas from Soho's, wine from the Farmer's Market, Starbuck's ice cream (I had to drive forty-five miles to get it) and Godiva chocolate. I tried to glue my heart back together with all the foods I found reassuring, but none of it worked. I immersed myself in misery, and nothing helped make me feel better or seemed to matter.

But it was the chocolate that consoled me. I found sad solace in those dark, sweet morsels. I was never more than a few feet from chocolate at any given place in my house, office or car. I had it in every form—Hershey's Kisses, Godiva Chocolate Seashells and Truffles, miniature candy bars, chocolate mints, chocolate coffee and chocolate-covered nuts. I had frozen fudge bars and coffee ice cream laden with chunks of chocolate. I started my day with mocha coffee and ended it with a chocolate bubble bath, which actually left me smelling like chocolate and made me eat more of it before falling asleep.

All this changed when I discovered my eight-pound weight loss. You don't spend as many years as I did trying to lose weight and not get exuberant when it happens with no effort on your part. Food suddenly became important again—but in a different way. I needed to take a good look at what I had been eating that accomplished this marvelous feat. Besides the early morning exercise, there had to be something going on with what went in my mouth that had facilitated this.

Not only had Sadie made total chaos out of my rigid daily routines, she had also done so to my food world. I had been too busy with her to keep my stash of chocolate or other indulgent foods in the house. This alone caused a major drop in my daily calorie consumption. While contemplating my eight-pound weight loss, I learned that some unexpected events certainly had made a dent in my eating binges. There were days I'd hardly eaten anything at all due to some unforeseen and completely unexpected dog-related mishap, especially on those mornings when I didn't know if I was yet fully awake or still asleep, including:

1. Using the same spoon in my coffee that I'd used to mix the dog food.
2. Having to clean up a dog "accident" just before trying to eat.
3. Finding a dog hair on my plate.
4. Catching her taking a bite from my plate when I'd left it on the edge of the coffee table.
5. Dropping food on the floor—gone in five seconds.
6. Taking the dog vitamin instead of my own.
7. Putting my cereal bowl on the floor by mistake and eating a spoonful of dog food instead.
8. Realizing I'd added puppy chow to my omelet instead of green peppers.
9. Leaving my food while taking her out to pee; she always beat me to it coming back in.
10. Burning my eggs while attending to some urgent dog need.

These occurrences did play a role in my unintentional and newly restricted calorie intake, thus dropping my weight, but this was only the beginning. Being able to eat any food at all would soon become a challenge.

Every diet I was ever on was about not eating certain things. All living creatures must eat to sustain themselves and to survive against predators. I never understood that "survival of the fittest" deal until Sadie slid into my kitchen on all four paws. After all, there hadn't been anyone else in the house to compete with for food. When I went to the refrigerator and everything was eaten, I knew who to blame, and it was always me. The human species is the only one consumed with NOT eating and, conversely, the only species with a serious obesity problem. Dogs not only eat *everything;* they eat *anything.*

Sadie's vet had strongly advised against giving her a taste of people food. Once she had a taste for it, he warned, I would be subjected to a lifetime of begging. I wondered how valid this information was because this dog seemed to know exactly what she wanted before she even had a tiny morsel of my food. How could he explain her demanding the last slice of pizza on that sleepless first night? She didn't need a taste to know that she wanted it . . . and everything else that I had that smelled even remotely like something she would enjoy. The appearance of food brought on endless barking, jumping and begging. She seemed to be born with this innate ability to beg for food she wasn't supposed to have. But the positive, if not miraculous, side of this was that it was usually food that I was not supposed to have either. Nonetheless, old habits die hard, and during those initial weeks with her I tried every possible diversion to keep her from knowing that I was eating.

The little black-as-licorice nose that had been so endearing to me in the first moments of meeting her became my nemesis. Forget the simple pleasures of a snack of popcorn or chips and dip. Her nose was as keen as burglar alarms in the rare painting room of a major museum. She could smell food from any corner of the house. If she was in the backyard and got a whiff of something coming from the kitchen exhaust fan, she'd dash into the kitchen, sniffing right to the source. The sound of unwrapping a chocolate bar always brought her running. If you've ever been at the beach and had sea-gulls jealously peering at you—watching for any scrap of food that you might drop—you have only a slight idea of what Sadie was like. All eight pounds of her were a quivering, ready alert to the slightest crumb, the faintest aroma or the smallest sound that might signal the presence of food.

I'd bought her a set of nice stainless steel bowls for food and water, which sat on a vinyl place mat on the kitchen floor. I'd been confident that she'd eat her dog food, I'd eat my people food, and harmony would ensue. I couldn't have been more wrong, and she took every opportunity to let me know it in the weeks that followed. I had no idea what a challenge even a simple meal would become with Sadie in the house. All of my former self-imposed food restrictions were nothing compared to the food fight that developed between us. It was war.

Sadie made eating even the smallest meal or snack totally impossible. She wanted everything. *Why oh why,* I asked myself, *had I given her ice cubes that first night?* I couldn't even fix a glass of ice water without her barking for "cubes." She usually gave me about ten seconds before the entreaties began and got louder as I attempted to ignore them.

During that despondent winter before Sadie arrived, food had never lasted long in my house. A lot of it was takeout, which, we all know, must be eaten immediately because it won't taste as good later on. Ingredients to actually make anything healthy, including fresh vegetables, made no appearances in my refrigerator that winter. When I started to backslide with eating, I went the entire distance. When Sadie arrived, I went from food overindulgence to near famine almost overnight.

Breakfast was out of the question. She'd hop out of bed with me and follow me to the kitchen. Initially, I'd put the coffee on and rummage around for something to eat after I prepared her food. While she greeted her food in a happy manner, she soon abandoned it when the prospect of something better appeared. No matter what I tried to eat, she wanted it. Even looking in the refrigerator was impossible. She'd leap at the shelves when I opened the door, knocking things off the racks and out of my hands. Once the refrigerator was opened, it was as if she thought she was on *Let's Make a Deal,* and door number three with all its riches was there for her taking.

Even before she began sleeping with me, the slim window of opportunity I had to grab something before descending to the basement to release her from her crate was way too brief. I'd reach blindly in the fridge and grab the first item my hand encountered. The taste of a cold egg roll or sushi before you've even had one cup of coffee is not a pleasant experience. And it didn't matter anyway because whatever I had managed to scarf down on the way to the basement, she'd smell on my hand or breath, and it triggered a renewed din of barking, licking and jumping. It simply was not worth the trouble.

However, there were two more meals to consider before I could go to bed hungry. Lunch had once been an opportunity to go out with friends. This was over; I had to take Sadie out. So I'd walk home, and her jovial little self would tumble out of the crate, and off we'd go. We developed a pattern of walking a mile each day at lunch; one half mile from our street to the bridge, and a half mile back. Unlike our brisk morning walks, our lunchtime walks were her opportunity to sniff the entire route, stare at boats on the river and in general just delay my attempts to get anything to eat. Usually my stomach was grumbling the entire walk.

Once back at the house, the food struggle would begin anew. Previously, I'd enjoyed eating lunch as I watched the noon news. This too was over. Sadie'd jump on my lap, often spilling whatever it was I was trying to eat on both the sofa and my clothes. Her food was in her dish and ready for consumption, but she didn't want it. She was ready at all times to pounce on whatever I was trying to eat. There we were, at a standoff.

My only recourse was to breeze through the capitol cafeteria, pick up something and eat it on the walk home. This was no easy task: I was always carrying a briefcase, and sometimes an umbrella, cell phone and purse. Most of whatever I had selected ended up on the ground (often eaten by Sadie as we ambled by it during her noontime walk) or on me (also eaten by Sadie as she licked the stains on my clothes). This plan was soon scrapped when my dry cleaning bill got too high, and I could no longer take the questioning looks when I'd come back from lunch wearing different clothes.

I also tried the cafeteria as a solution for my dinner dilemma. But since it closed at 2:00 P.M., I'd have to go through the cafeteria once again on my way back from lunch. Overcoming the quizzical stares from the cafeteria staff, who obviously were thinking I certainly didn't need two lunches, was only one of the problems this solution presented. Food purchased from an institutional cafeteria has questionable quality at its peak, and I was buying it for dinner at least three hours before I would eat it. It was just barely better than eating nothing at all by the time I'd consume it for dinner.

I tried taking the Styrofoam containers of my room-temperature cafeteria food home after work and eating in the kitchen before getting Sadie out of her crate. But she was always alerted to my arrival when I turned off the security alarm. I simply couldn't eat with all that barking and banging going on in the crate a floor beneath me. Eating this food after she was out of the crate at a normal dinnertime just didn't work. She wanted it and would race around the kitchen island jumping on me. It got worse after I struggled through a few dinners and allowed her to lick the Styrofoam containers. There was no more guessing as to what was in these containers. Now she knew it was edible, and she wasn't content with traces of leftovers. She wanted to have all of it. So I started eating room-temperature institutional food at my desk before walking home. This soon proved to be futile as well. I only worked until 4:00 P.M. and was hungry before I even got home, and by 7:00 P.M. I was starving again.

Another solution I tried was to go home and, after a couple of hours, hop in my car and go to a drive-through and eat in the car on the way back home. I could never accomplish this without spilling something on myself, which Sadie would inevitably smell as I got her out of her crate, thus causing more jumping and licking. During one of these scenes, she got so excited by some blue cheese dressing that my new Rayure blouse ended up with little teeth holes in it. Besides the blouse costing more than the dog and all her possessions, what really got me mad was that I was still hungry.

Some days, I'd just eat a huge lunch hoping to avoid the evening meal problem altogether. This, too, had serious consequences. First of all, it was extremely difficult to maintain any type of mental acuity, sometimes even consciousness, following these lunchtime gastronomical extravagances. To my extreme embarrassment, a transcript arrived one day for a deposition that I didn't even remember attending. It was only apparent that I had been there because the court reporter noted my appearance in the beginning of the transcript; however, I had not asked a single question. I was relieved when the case settled soon after that, and I didn't have to face the other attorneys who were present to find out if I'd slept through the entire proceeding.

After these huge lunches, I felt bloated, and my clothes fit so tightly that I always ended the day with some serious welts around my waist that were both unsightly and uncomfortable. And by bed-time, I was plain famished, if not nursing the beginning of a headache.

I tried sneaking to the kitchen without her noticing, but Sadie followed me everywhere. She could appear to be in the deepest of sleeps, somewhere off in dog delicatessen dreams, but the moment I put one leg on the floor, she was up. I was foolish enough to try eating some ice cream in bed one night. She ran up and down my legs and pounced on my bowl. Not only did I not get one bite dur-ing the fracas, but chocolate ice cream was smeared everywhere, and I had to change my sheets.

Of course, I had the option of eating my meals out, sitting down at a restaurant, but this also was an untenable solution. The first hurdle was just leaving Sadie at home. She seemed to have an understanding that I had to go to work, thus she had to be left alone in her crate, but dashing home at noon and only taking the necessary time to take her for a bathroom break was unacceptable to her. Even more egregious was my leaving her again in the evening. She'd bite my clothes as I attempted to change them, often ruining my panty hose. Then she would put her head down, while turning her eyes up toward me in the saddest, most forlorn manner.

And when I put her in the crate . . . well, she delivered her final admonishment to me without even a bark.

She never rebelled and refused to go. Quite the opposite; she'd hang her head, go down the steps slowly, take her paw and bat open the door to her crate and go in ever so slowly. Her last attempt to get me to stay home was to flop on her mattress and emit a huge sigh. I just couldn't leave her, even if it meant missing a good dinner. We might have gotten off to a rocky start and were still finding our way together, but I loved her now, and she meant everything to me.

There were two things that alerted Sadie to food and me eating. The most obvious one was smell. If a food item had any odor that Sadie detected as something good to eat, I was licked in more ways than one. The other was sound. She could hear the refrigerator door open from anywhere in the house. Even at her young puppy stage, she somehow knew to associate the sound of packages opening—cellophane in particular—with food, and was ready for action.

So, I reasoned, if I only ate food that was quiet and didn't smell good, I might not be prohibited from eating in my own home. I would be able to freely go into my kitchen and get something to eat and maybe even eat it at my breakfast room table.

I began to examine food packaging. I searched up and down supermarket aisles looking for things in packages that wouldn't make noise. This proved to be a much bigger problem than I'd imagined. Almost everything is packaged in something that rustles, pops, squeaks, crunches or requires a can opener, which to Sadie immediately signals "food is on the way." Initially, I was particularly interested in items that would satisfy my hunger before bed, and I searched for perfect late-night snack items.

If you aren't having great sex before falling asleep, the next best thing is a cold turkey sandwich on rye with lettuce, onion, pickles and brown mustard. Almost every ingredient of this longed-for pleasure was beyond my acquisition because of the noise involved in procuring them. The sad fact is that when the house is totally quiet, the sounds emitted opening these packages are greatly amplified, easily arousing the food patrol, even when she was in the basement.

I carefully scanned supermarket shelves for items that would meet my taste criteria, which was growing smaller as my hunger increased. Basically, if it was edible and in a container that would open silently, it was going into my cart. Because they don't allow you to test this feature of the food package in the store, I bought endless items that seemed appropriate and took them home to test their noise level as they were being opened.

Things in a jar seemed a safe bet. How noisy can it be getting a jar lid off? I was wrong. Professional wrestlers must put the lids on jars of food products these days. I couldn't find one jar that didn't need to be banged on the sink counter to be opened, thus alerting Sadie that something was going on in the kitchen and, of course, it could only mean food.

Cereal? Out of the question. It might have been possible if the inner sealed bag wasn't so unbelievably noisy, that is, if tearing the cardboard zipper of the box top was possible without her hearing it. Anything frozen was out because it would have to be microwaved, and the sound of the microwave alarm always brought her immediately into the kitchen. I even considered letting a frozen dinner thaw on the kitchen island and eating it at room temperature. My desperation was deepening.

In my previous diet-crazed life, I used to give my elderly neighbor across the street any perishable food when I was going out of town for a business trip. Depending on what diet I was employing at the time, she'd often seem puzzled at some of my offerings. I remember giving her about three dozen grapefruits and several pounds of Canadian bacon. Another time it was a half gallon of egg whites and a dozen green peppers. But now as I began showing up on a regular basis with all sorts of items in open packages that had not even been tasted, she began to look at me strangely. At first, I just couldn't bring myself to tell her what was really going on. So I made up excuses. The flimsier my excuses became the stranger the looks I got.

One day I ventured across the street with a very noisy bag of tortilla chips. All right, I did manage to eat a handful of chips on my way over, and they were so good I considered turning around and keeping them in my car. "These were too salty." (Do they make unsalty tortilla chips?) I'd been quite excited with a box of Little Debbie Cakes in a soft cardboard box. To my huge dismay they were individually wrapped in noisy cellophane wrappers. "I thought these were something else." (I couldn't see the picture on the package?) My one attempt at something good for me was a dozen organic eggs. Unfortunately, they were in a cellophane-wrapped Styrofoam container that squeaked loudly when opened. "These are from the wrong kind of chicken." That was the one that did me in, and I had to confess what was going on. Virginia laughed at me and told everyone on her side of the street. From then on, I had an audience when I trekked across the street with rejected food.

I tried putting Sadie out in the backyard so I could sneak into the kitchen and eat. She loved the backyard—but, you guessed it, only when I was there; otherwise she went into hysterical bark mode. I simply had to bring her in to avoid my neighbors calling the police. I tried putting a sandwich in my pocket to eat while she was absorbed on her walk. Not only did it fall apart as I tried to get it out, but she refused to move from the sidewalk until every morsel was gone.

I tried eating at the same time as she did. I'd pop something in the microwave while I prepared her food. She would sit smack in front of the microwave sniffing the air. When I removed my food, I'd place her bowl on the floor, attempting to trick her into thinking she was getting the same thing. She didn't buy it for a minute and jumped on me and howled, wanting what I had. So I microwaved her food right along with mine. This was successful only for Sadie. She loved her food warm and wolfed it down before I even got to my second bite, which tasted like her food smelled. I tried this several times, but no matter how good the Lean Cuisine package looked, when it smelled like Sadie's food, I lost my appetite for it. I actually briefly considered eating her food. I did eat one of her snacks and found it acceptable, but I didn't think I could live on them. Here was this darling little food demon enjoying meals *and* snacks, while I was barely getting enough calories for energy to stay awake all afternoon.

The only alternative I could think of that I had not tried was to just get earplugs (for me—I didn't think they made them for dogs) and put her in the crate while I ate and tried to ignore her barking. This never got beyond the planning stages. If you think moms are good at making you feel guilty, they're rank amateurs compared to a dog. I simply couldn't bring myself to do it.

So I set about making a list of all the foods that were odor free, as well as the ones I'd discovered in noiseless packages. I narrowed down the list to the ones I thought I could survive on. This was no easy task. If something met one of the criteria, it failed the other. As I accumulated entries for my list, I noticed an interesting pattern evolving. Most of these foods were healthy and good for me compared to the ones I tried to "sneak eat" away from Sadie. Here was another way I was losing weight. These foods not only were nutritious, they were low calorie. Sure, they might not be the tastiest or anywhere near gourmet quality, but in my quest for slimness, I had eaten a lot worse in the past.

Remember, if you think your dog shouldn't be eating something, then you probably shouldn't be eating it either. Foods like pizza, chocolate and ice cream are good examples. Your dog shouldn't eat these things, and if you want to get slim, you shouldn't either, at least not on a regular basis.

I began to appreciate Sadie's obsession with food and saw it as a positive means of reinforcement for my diet. There are human equivalents to this canine food cop. They're called personal chefs and can cost hundreds of dollars a week. You pay them to come to your home and place only certain foods in your refrigerator. They make daily visits to inspect the inventory in your refrigerator, and you have to pay them even more if there are unauthorized foods in there or you have eaten foods prematurely. In the worst of cases, which more than likely I would have qualified for, they don't allow you to keep any food in the house and deliver your daily calorie allowance meal by meal. This gold service can cost you over a thousand dollars a week.

I realized how lucky I was. I had a $40 dog doing it for me, and it wasn't costing me a thing except a few vet bills and her food and treats—a very small price to pay. In fact, I was realizing what a great bargain Sadie was in this overall diet and exercise scheme. I had surely spent thousands of dollars on weekly magazines touting various diet schemes, let alone all the foods needed to implement the plans. Each week had brought a new round of magazines and foods to buy, prepare and eat. Sadie's methods remained constant; there were no changes in her plans when it came to food. Also, I'd never felt better about trying to lose weight. Personal trainers I'd had in the past were always upbeat and had a good attitude, but Sadie had the best outlook of any person I had ever known—and she didn't criticize my efforts; she only wanted to eat my food.

So it was that quiet foods that didn't emit tempting aromas began to compose my daily diet. If they were tasteless or unimaginative, it didn't matter. It beat trying to walk or drive while eating, falling asleep at my desk or going to bed hungry with a headache. I was playing a meal-by-meal game trying to outwit this little food cop, and in the process I was getting thinner and laughing a whole lot more.

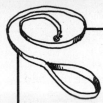

Dog Diet

DISCOVERIES

1. If it goes into your dog's mouth, it doesn't go on your waistline!

2. Remember, if something isn't good for your dog, it probably isn't good for you either.

3. Letting your dog control your calorie intake beats counting and detailing your daily diet.

4. Your dog is the best bet to getting you back into those old jeans.

5. Dogs make the best personal trainers.

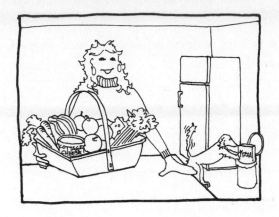

CHAPTER FOUR

Foolproof Foods

(If it's quiet and doesn't smell good . . . quick, eat it!)

*T*hings were definitely looking up in my life now, and I gave credit for much of that to Sadie. Despite the food struggles and the lack of sleep that had seemed unbearable, I was twelve pounds lighter and had a better attitude than I'd had all winter, or in years for that matter. We were settling into a comfortable, albeit somewhat irregular, routine. Our walking program kept me busy and had renewed my interest in keeping the numbers on the scale going down. But the hit-and-miss or, more accurately, grab-and-gobble, system I was forced to use to get anything to eat had to change.

My past failures with dieting had at least taught me that all weight-loss plans have two components: an eating plan and an exercise plan. I decided to call the new exercise regimen and eating deprivation that Sadie had devised for me the Dog Diet. Like all other diet schemes, it too would need an eating plan. I needed to work on developing a selection of foods that met the criteria that would allow me to eat both alone and in front of her, those being:

1. Packaged food that can be removed from its container relatively quietly and eaten without audible crunches or other noise.
2. Food that doesn't have a tantalizing aroma.

I also began to add foods to the list that Sadie didn't like, even though, initially, the only one I'd discovered was olives. As I had done with all my other diets, when I first started trying to put this food plan together, I wanted to see if I could come up with one of the "have-my-cake-and-eat-it-too" methods I'd hung on to in the past. I briefly considered the following solutions:

1. Putting a microwave in my garage.
2. Installing a small kitchen on the third floor of the house—far from the basement.
3. Keeping a supply of tuna and a can opener in my office.
4. Ordering a supply of military rations to keep in my bedroom.
5. Using the roof of my porch located outside my bedroom for food storage.

Some of these were too expensive, and some were too ridiculous. What would the capitol police think as they watched me sneak out to my garage in the middle of the night? How would my clients react to their letters smelling like tuna fish?

No, it was apparent that I needed to develop a diet that we both could live with. It didn't seem like it would be too difficult to create a new eating routine considering all the hundreds of food combinations I'd created in the past. I thought of the countless shopping trips for items such as seaweed, wheatgrass or the flaxseed that needed to be ground up and ruined my coffee grinder. I'd choked down numerous chalky-tasting milkshakes, sautéed instead of fried and lived on portion-control frozen dinners that tasted like their cardboard containers instead of the delicious meals pictured on the box. I'd spent hours in various markets reading labels and swallowed hundreds of fat burners, though the only thing they ever seemed to burn was my money. I was ready to create a rational and cost-effective eating plan that would work.

I calculated that, factoring in the cost of the instructional materials, I'd paid as much as $47 a pound to lose weight with past diets. I was shocked by this realization. I couldn't remember ever purchasing a food that cost this much. This calculation didn't even take into account the few measly pounds I'd managed to lose in a week at more than one pricey spa. Think about it: if you go to a spa that costs $2,000 a week (been there, done that), and you lose the "safe" two pounds recommended in a week's time, you have paid $1,000 for each of those pounds. Then you go home, and it costs you under $5 for one carton of Ben and Jerry's New York Super Fudge Chunk ice cream as your reward, and you gain it all back.

One program that I'd found easy to live with because it allowed me to eat six times a day required a $300 start-up kit. The kit consisted of tasteless milkshakes, fat calipers I never did learn how to use, a video I couldn't keep up with and a journal that wasn't as good as the notebook I kept on my own.

All of the diets I'd been on came with their own stringent list of foods that you could eat, and an equally rigid list of ones that you couldn't eat. I reviewed the foods and matched them with my new criteria, and chose cottage cheese as my first Dog Diet delicacy. Cottage cheese is almost the perfect food. It comes in a low-fat version, it's inexpensive, has no delicious aroma, and the packaging and the food itself are quiet. The cottage cheese test was great at first.

Initially I thought that I might be able to live solely on cottage cheese. I ate cottage cheese with olives, cottage cheese with fresh fruit and cottage cheese with applesauce and apple butter. I had it for breakfast with salsa, for lunch with cayenne pepper, for dinner with olives. Soon, though, I was sick of it. Sadie's vet had also told me a little cottage cheese was good for her. Sadie didn't know the meaning of a "little bit," and after that first serving, she was right there each time the container came out of the refrigerator.

I set out to expand the list with foods that met the two criteria and any other food I discovered that she didn't like. These foods would hopefully be "stand alone" foods like the cottage cheese, foods you could make a meal out of with nothing else and that required little preparation. The least amount of time I had to spend in the kitchen the better, because any kitchen activity brought Sadie to investigate. Additionally, with all the time I now spent taking care of Sadie, anything that saved a few minutes was appreciated.

Then I would move on to phase 2 of the Dog Diet and create some actual meals by combining these foods. They would be perfect, and maybe I could even serve them to company if I ever had a date again. My intention was to have a large enough selection of foods that it would be a snap to put together a meal in mere minutes. Well, the best-laid plans are often eaten by the dog.

It proved more difficult than I imagined. Even though it was not an extremely short list, none of the food items seemed to go together in quite the way I expected. How long can you exist on cold hard-boiled eggs and uncooked broccoli? Or worse, cold black beans and yogurt?

I found myself on the all-raw-food diet I'd previously purchased a book about and never got around to actually trying. Most of the foods had to be eaten raw because cooking brought out their enticing aromas. Even warming them up in the microwave was impossible because Sadie knew that the sound of the timer alarm meant food. A steady diet of raw food was less satisfying than eating nothing at all.

Most diets advocate eating at specific times, the number of times you eat a day and a time after which you absolutely cannot eat anything at all. It's usually recommended that you also eat slowly, chew your food thoughtfully and give your brain twenty minutes to let your stomach know that it has eaten. How this could be done with some of the diet foods that tasted so bad they were almost impossible to swallow was beyond me.

None of these admonishments became part of the Dog Diet. No, I didn't even consider any of them when designing my eating plan. As a matter of fact, eating at any time at all was such an accomplishment that it didn't matter when I was able to ingest something. Eating slowly was out of the question. How can you eat slowly when at any minute the canine food terminator might appear? In fact, I recommend you learn to eat as quickly as possible, scarfing down your food as fast as you can before your dog has a clue that you're eating—that is, if you don't want to share it.

Putting these foods together became quite a predicament. I plunged right in though, and although my menus were limited, I was surviving and spending a lot less money on food than I had before Sadie arrived. Below is the list of foods, in no particular order, except maybe the order they were discovered in (I wasn't too picky by this time as you'll see). I called them "Foolproof Foods," because they were intended to fool Sadie and serve as proof to me that I *could* eat despite her efforts, and that I would continue to lose weight.

Foolproof Foods

Beverages

Water: Water soon became almost my sole beverage. It was easy to get a glass of ice water and throw a few ice cubes in Sadie's bowl. There were no pop can tabs that sparked her curiosity and made her

jump on me for a taste. During one
of my previous diets, I had learned
that our bodies burns up forty extra
calories just to warm up the ice
water. Whether this is true or not,
I had no idea, but I *did* know that
drinking lots of water was good for
me and that water had no calories. I
started squirting a little lime juice from
one of those plastic limes into my water to
give it some taste. A plastic lime has no odor and doesn't make
noise, so it was perfect.

Chill your water glass in the freezer along with a slice of lime or lemon. It adds a special touch to drinking ice water. You can turn this into a tasty glass of faux champagne by adding some ginger ale to the ice water.

Coffee: Coffee was my salvation during those early days of little
sleep. I simply never considered giving it up and was fortunate that
the smell of coffee did nothing for Sadie. She simply paid no attention to my coffee drinking, and this was great.

Unprocessed Foods

This list does include some foods that are noisy to eat, but to my
utter delight, I discovered most of them were foods that Sadie just
didn't like. Offering a small bite of any of these foods was like
magic. She'd just give it a few licks and leave it—and me—alone.
I've checked this out with other dog "moms" who confirm that
their dogs also turned their tails and ran when given vegetables or
fruit. What a boon to my list as these items are a staple for any
weight-loss regimen.

(I would note here, however, that as time went on, Sadie started to like certain fruits and vegetables, and I've since learned that they are very good for dogs. Green beans and cooked potatoes became a favorite, and I never minded sharing them with her. Check with your vet and other dog parents and you will find lots of tips for feeding your dog fresh vegetables and fruit.)

Almonds	Cucumbers	Pears
Apples	Dried cranberries	Plums
Arugula and	Ginger	Potatoes
other greens	Grapefruit/oranges	Radishes
Beets	Green beans	Raspberries
Blueberries	Green onions	Sprouts
Broccoli	Green, red, or	Strawberries
Cabbage—green	yellow peppers	Sugar snap peas
and red	Hard-boiled eggs	in shell
Carrots	Jicama	Turnips
Cauliflower	Kiwifruit	Watermelon
Celery	Lettuce	Yams
Cherry Tomatoes	Mangoes	Yellow squash
Cilantro	Mushrooms	Zucchini

Fresh, raw green beans actually aren't that bad. You can even add them to a salad. However, the small cans with the pull-tab tops can also be used. With practice you will be able to open these cans almost silently. This also works for any other vegetable in pull-tab cans except corn. Corn has a strong aroma and immediately got Sadie's attention. She also liked peas, but a dog-owning neighbor told me that a few peas were good for dogs. I had this confirmed by the vet, and, of course, a few peas soon progressed to a can for her and a can for me. Hey, eating an entire can of peas was nothing compared to eating an entire pizza or pint of ice cream.

Raw potatoes don't sound very appetizing, although with salt and garlic pepper, they're not too bad, and I knew enough about nutrition to realize I needed potassium in my diet. At one extreme diet spa I went to, our daily happy hour consisted of "cocktails" of water that potatoes had soaked in overnight. The theory was, and at least they made it sound plausible enough for numerous women like me to shell out big bucks for a week of these sorts of practices, that the potassium from the potatoes leached into the water overnight. We got all the benefit of the potatoes, none of the carbs and none of the calories. For months following my stay at this place, I had pitchers of water in my refrigerator with potatoes in them. On a few occasions, I forgot this and offered the water to company.

When choosing lettuce, get different varieties. If possible get organic salad greens to which you can add romaine, and my favorite, arugula. The prepackaged salad mixes are nice as well. Fresh dill is a great flavor enhancer to salad as are other fresh herbs.

If you have space for a garden, or even a few container plants, homegrown herbs and vegetables are great additions to your meals. Rosemary will grow all winter even in cold climates. Another alternative is a windowsill herb garden. I grow hot peppers and save the seeds for flavoring.

Try to find unusual fruits. I love pomegranates, passion fruit, star fruit, Asian pears and others. These can make a lovely garnish on a plate, or be blended into a great sweet sauce with the addition of a little honey.
(See recipe section.)

Their pained expressions confirmed my own suspicions, not only about the taste of this water, but my own sanity to have paid money to indulge in such silly practices and the validity of the spa's claim concerning this.

Processed Foods

Applesauce	Mandarin oranges,	Refried beans
Apple butter	canned	Ricotta cheese
Black beans	Mayonnaise	Salad dressings
Brown rice	Mustard	Salsa
Chutney	Olives	Sour cream
Cottage cheese	Pasta (any kind)	Sun-dried tomatoes
Dried spices	Pickled	Tomatoes, canned
Hot, pickled	cauliflower	Whole-wheat
vegetables	Pickles	tortillas
Hot sauces	Red pepper spread	Yogurt

Discovering the whole-wheat tortillas was the turning point that made me believe that being able to eat normally would return to my world (of course, my overindulgent eating prior to Sadie's watch had certainly not been close to normal). These tortillas were my salvation. Any of the above ingredients could be wrapped in the tortilla, and with a squirt of mustard, I had a sandwich. The best part of these wonderful low-carb tortillas was that Sadie would have nothing to do with them. After several offerings of the tortilla met with rejection, I was free to enjoy it. She'd look at it and turn around and leave the kitchen. It had so

Any good-flavored, low-fat salad dressing can be used in a variety of ways. Experiment making your own. Whisk some lemon or lime into olive oil, add fresh ground pepper and drizzle it over vegetables or salads for a tasty experience.

many excellent qualities, including that it came in a large size that had only 80 calories! It also had 14 grams of fiber, another essential element in weight loss as I'd learned in the past, no cholesterol, 3 grams of fat, and 8 grams of protein. It quickly became my favorite food, and I ate everything wrapped in one of them. As Sadie sat and just looked at me, the pleasure I experienced munching on a tortilla filled with green peppers, lettuce, cucumbers and cherry tomatoes was indescribable!

And so I began the task of fashioning meals from these ingredients. While challenging, it was not impossible. The cold bean burrito became the staple of my diet. Heating refried beans in the microwave brought Sadie's usual reaction to possibly appealing food, so I simply ate them cold. I'd spread about a half cup of the beans over the tortilla, add lettuce and salsa, and enjoy. I was getting important nutrients here, they weren't tasty enough to encourage me to a second helping, and they were easy. I could prepare these ahead of time and leave them in the refrigerator. As a special treat, I'd add a little dollop of sour cream. I always felt satiated after eating one.

The bean burrito was a universal meal and could be served for breakfast, lunch or dinner. I soon became quite creative, adding cold brown rice and cherry tomatoes, as well as other ingredients from my list. Let your imagination be your guide and the combinations are plentiful. One of my favorite burritos includes fresh cilantro, arugula, salsa and onions.

I was soon eating all of these foods just as easily as I'd eaten the gluttonous foods of my past. The one indulgence I didn't give up was chocolate, although my consumption was quite limited. Sadie ran into the kitchen if she heard me opening a chocolate bar. But I'd been told by yet another dog parent that chocolate was toxic for dogs. I *couldn't* give it to her . . . it would harm her. So I just savored my occasional bite of chocolate, and nothing she did caused this enjoyment to ebb! I no longer concealed chocolate all over the house, but kept a small supply in the refrigerator crisper. Just knowing that this tiny shred of my former life was still available to me was a pleasant feeling.

In no time, the Dog Diet was a routine part of my life. Did I still long for my old eating habits? You bet I did. Each time I went to the supermarket, I searched for items to add to my food list. The list didn't expand much, but my methods for handling Sadie did. I reasoned that if some of my human food was good for her, then I could start sharing meals with her. I decided to check out my hypothesis with her vet. I'm not sure that he'd ever been asked, "Can my dog and I eat the same food?" but he handled it expertly.

Dr. Settee gave me a list, albeit short, of things that would be good for Sadie to eat along with me. It consisted of:

- Rice
- Yogurt
- Cottage cheese
- Hard-boiled eggs
- Tuna (packed in water)

My disappointment was profound. Except for the tuna, these items were already part of my daily diet and offered none of the appetizing diversions I had envisioned! Driving to the vet, I had imagined being able to order a deluxe pizza once again and slipping a piece or two in Sadie's bowl as I munched away blissfully. Realizing this was probably never going to happen, I took comfort in the appearance of tuna on the list and began instantly thinking of the many concoctions I could create with its addition to my food list.

He did give me one glimmer of hope. Ice cream could return to my diet. While he advised against giving Sadie ice cream, and I already knew what her reaction was when I tried to eat it, he did tell me about a form of dog ice cream. There was an item on the market called "Frosty Paws," a nondairy form of ice cream completely good for dogs. He suggested I give this a try. She could have her ice cream, and I would have mine!

I was so enthused that I went straight from the vet's office to the supermarket. Dismayed that I couldn't find the Frosty Paws, I asked the manager where they were. He looked at me like I was out of my mind and assured me that if such a thing existed, it would be quite a while before it ever came to Charleston. Undaunted, I went to a larger store, by this time almost running to the ice-cream freezer, scanned the many shelves, and there they were! I opened the freezer and grabbed two packages of the brightly colored boxes with a happy white dog on them. I snatched two pints of Ben and Jerry's New York Super Fudge Chunk for myself. I hadn't had any such delicacy during the many weeks since Sadie's arrival. It took all the restraint I had not to open the carton and take a lick of it while I was waiting in line.

I implemented my experiment as soon as we got home. Throwing the extra containers in the freezer, I ripped one of the Frosty Paws out of the box and placed it on the floor for Sadie as I tore the lid off my own ice cream. Even if this didn't work out, I'd be able to get in a few fast bites before she rejected her doggy version of this treat.

Miraculous! She was totally engrossed in her little cup of dog ice cream, and I was happily eating my own chocolate decadence. Funny thing, though, I only wanted a few spoonfuls. When Sadie was finished devouring her treat, I too was done with mine, and placed the remainder in the freezer. If I had still been keeping my diet journal, this would have been the first entry where I could note that I had *not* eaten the entire container! No longer did I need the comfort of food; Sadie was my comfort, and she was completely calorie free.

I should probably say something here about "Forbidden Foods," which every diet I'd ever played around with had a list of. However, the book would be endless, so I won't go into that in detail. Almost anything that's not on the Foolproof Foods lists was forbidden, not by my standards, but Sadie's. The one substance that deserves a cautionary warning is alcohol.

I didn't even try to have any wine in the house after one episode when I popped the cork only to have a startled Sadie leap right at the bottle I was holding, knocking it to the floor. It was chaos, holding Sadie back from lapping up the wine as I tried to mop it up. I didn't want to waste any more wine on the kitchen floor, but I quickly came to my senses regarding this libation anyway. How on earth would I ever be able to get up and take this dog out if I had a hangover? It would be unbearable! Given my sleep-deprived state at the time, being lulled to dreamland in a warm, fuzzy, wine haze was a tempting idea, but the thought of my mornings being any worse than they actually were stopped me dead in my tracks.

Combining ingredients for meals became intriguing. I wasn't starving, I still had energy to exercise, and I was continuing to lose weight. All of those diets with rigid guidelines of what must be eaten when and with what were history. I simply put together items from the foods on hand that might be good together, and I had a meal—a meal that required little if any cooking. And when I did cook, it was most often something that I could share with Sadie or that she had no taste for. I was ready for food each morning as Sadie and I ran into the house from our exercise session. I wasn't dreaming of bacon and eggs anymore, and my new foods were becoming more palatable. Beginning with breakfast, I developed a number of low-calorie, healthy, easy-to-fix meals.

Breakfast

- **Bean Burrito:** Take one large La Tortilla whole-wheat tortilla. Spread one-half cup of refried beans on it. I use the black beans. They have many great nutritional qualities that I can't remember, but I also like their taste better! Add lettuce and salsa. Roll this up, cut in half. These can also be made the night before if you want to save time in the morning for extra walking.
- **Cottage Cheese and Fruit:** Use one-half cup of your favorite cottage cheese, add any fruit you have on hand and enjoy.
- **Hard-boiled Egg and Yogurt:** You can either boil the eggs the night before and keep them in the fridge or cook them that morning. This is a meal you can share with your dog.
- **Leftovers:** Any cold leftovers from the night before will work just fine for breakfast.
- **Yogurt and Cottage Cheese:** Mixing these two together makes a great breakfast.
- **Yogurt and Fruit**

If you're shaking your head and thinking these breakfasts are bland, think again. What did sausage and eggs ever do for you? These new breakfasts allowed me to eat in peace, which I had come to place a huge value on. Being able to eat anything in the mornings was such a privilege! Any habitual dieter can tell just by looking at this list that these foods are good for you. Okay, I didn't say they were deliciously good, just good for you, and they aren't the worst thing you or I ever put in our mouths in order to take inches off our waists. In fact, they were downright gourmet meals compared to the myriad of diet shakes I had forced down in the past! And here's the deal: if you still feel you need those shakes, and they make you feel like you're performing some kind of contrition for a secret eating sin the night before, go for it. Sadie never found herself attracted to even one diet shake, and your dog probably won't either.

Lunch and dinner came together much like the breakfast. I found that all of these foods could be eaten for any meal. The addition of tuna fish seemed to infinitely increase my choices. After our mile walk, we were now able to eat lunch together. Lunches no longer brought on a feeling of deprivation or that I was missing out by not going out to lunch with my friends. There was no way sitting in a restaurant and ordering anything on the menu could compare to this . . . could it?

Lunch

- **Bean Buritto:** These can be prepared the same as for breakfast, but you might want to add some additional lettuce and vegetables.
- **Egg Salad Burrito:** Chop up a hard-boiled egg for yourself and one for your dog. Mix hers with her food, and while she is eating, mix some mayonnaise and mustard with yours.

Spread this on one of your tortillas, add lettuce, a dash of hot sauce for good measure, and there you have a fantastic lunch.

- **Grapefruit with Cottage Cheese:** You can also use any of the other fruits from the list that you have on hand. This also is a great breakfast. The citrus will give your taste buds a wake-up shock. Other favorite fruits with cottage cheese at lunch are blackberries, peaches and mandarin oranges.

- **Raw Vegetable Plate with Cottage Cheese:** Use any of the great vegetables on your list. My favorites soon became the red peppers, yellow squash, broccoli, jicama and celery. You can use a small amount of your salad dressing as a dip for the vegetables.

- **Salad:** I began having a BIG salad for lunch every day. For protein, I would add tuna, a hard-boiled egg or cottage cheese. I even began bringing a piece of chicken home from the cafeteria and was able to slip it into the salad undetected. Any dressing will do, and from my previous dieting quests, I already had my favorite low-calorie, low-fat ones. The salad should contain as many of the vegetables you have on hand as possible.

- **Salad in a Tortilla:** This is a great way to add fiber to your diet. The tortilla gives a sense of fullness that you just don't get from a plain salad. You can put some red pepper spread on the tortilla in place of salad dressing. It's fat free and spicy, adding a zesty taste to your lunch.

- **Tuna Salad:** The little pull-tab cans of white tuna are my favorite. Sadie, however, has no preference in tuna; she likes it all. So, after you open it and before adding mayonnaise, give your dog a little bit of it. A good tuna salad also has celery and onions, so chop those up and stir them in along with a hard-boiled egg if you like. Spread this on your tortilla, add lettuce, roll it up and cut in half. Advance preparation will give you more time to play with your dog at lunchtime. I found myself enjoying games of tennis ball retrieval during lunch more often when I had prepared my lunch ahead of time.

What surprised me most about eating these lunches was that I had great energy in the afternoons. No more half-asleep, postlunch work sessions, and no more thinking about food all afternoon.

During the formulation of these meals I discovered a time-saving way to have the main ingredients for most of my meals ready and waiting in the refrigerator. I call it the Salad Box. I had one of those large plastic storage containers, which turned out to be the perfect storage container for the many vegetables and lettuces I used to create my meals.

When I'd come home from the grocery store, I'd clean and cut the various vegetables into bite-size portions and place all of them in the container together with the cleaned and dried lettuces. That way each meal did not require so much preparation time. I just had to open the box and pick out what I wanted. Grab a handful of the mix, place it on a plate, and you have an instant salad. The only thing you have to add is fresh tomatoes and salad dressing if you want.

Take your time washing and preparing the

vegetables to go into the Salad Box. Experiment with different ways of slicing and chopping. The one kitchen item I use the most now has nothing to do with a special diet and is not electronic. I use a mandoline to cut and slice vegetables into different thicknesses and shapes. My salads and vegetables look more appealing, and it's an exercise for my creativity!

You'll find the Salad Box a marvelous way to breeze through meal preparation and be surprised at how fresh everything stays in the storage container (complete instructions for creating a Salad Box are on page 217).

Dinner can be anything you want! Remember, any of these meals can be interchanged for a different time of day. For example, during the hot summer months, I found myself enjoying cottage cheese and fruit for dinner, or a big salad with some cold chicken (requires some furtive maneuvering) and as time went on, cold salmon.

I discovered that I liked salmon for breakfast as well. I'd cook salmon for dinner and, miraculously, there was something about the smell of salmon cooking that seemed to repel, rather than attract, Sadie. Each of these little Dog Diet "discoveries" added a new dimension to my eating that improved the overall quality of my meals. For dinner I created a few special meals that you'll find delicious, low calorie and simple to prepare. And just in case you do get the opportunity to invite a date over for dinner, not only are these meals perfectly presentable, but your dog won't be begging at the table!

Dinner

- **Black Bean and Shrimp Salad:** Mix about a cup of small shrimp in a bowl with black beans, cilantro, green onions and black olives. You can use your favorite salad dressing or mix up your own concoction. This is also great with just a dash of Tabasco and a squirt of lime juice.

- **Chicken with Brown Rice:** This dish has absolutely no aroma at all if eaten cold, and it's not bad that way. This works very well wrapped in one of your tortillas. Again, sharing the rice with your dog might make heating it a viable option. Sadie never even suspects that she is missing out on chicken when I share the rice with her! I cut the chicken in cubes and mix it with the rice and salsa. A small salad completes this great dinner.

- **Cold Shrimp with Salad:** The great thing about shrimp is that you can purchase it already cooked! Sadie never even smells it or, if she does, she ignores it. I was thrilled to add shrimp to my diet. Make a big salad and add shrimp to it, or eat the shrimp separately with cocktail sauce. Add some black beans to your salad for a different taste plus added protein and fiber.

- **Romaine Lettuce Salad with Salmon:** For the salad, use about half a head of crisp romaine lettuce and add any of the vegetables from the list. The salmon can either be cooked and served warm on the lettuce or prepared ahead of time and served cold. Either way it's delicious. Here's a good way to prepare the salmon:

1. Turn your toaster oven or regular oven to broil.
2. Cover a small broiling pan with aluminum foil and spray with PAM or any other no-stick agent.
3. Sprinkle some Tony Chachere's Creole seasoning on the salmon.
4. Place under the broiler for the amount of time necessary to cook to your specifications (I usually set my oven timer for twenty minutes).

A 6-ounce serving of salmon makes a satisfying dinner. Save any leftovers for breakfast.

• **Shrimp with Rice and Vegetables:** You can use any of the vegetables in your Salad Box mixed with a cup of brown rice (precooked in your fridge) and a cup of small salad shrimp. If you're lucky enough to be able to heat it undetected, splendid! You can pacify your dog if you attempt this by giving her some of the rice. However, if heating it proves impossible, it works fine cold as well. Just mix it thoroughly with a few tablespoons of your favorite salad dressing, and it will be wonderful!

Dessert

I formulated a few desserts that are low in calories and healthy as well. Something always seems lacking if you don't have dessert with dinner. Even the most severe, food-restricted diets have something that masquerades as dessert. These Dog Diet desserts hit the spot, none of them requires extensive preparation, and they're all satisfying for your sweet tooth.

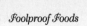

- **Fresh Fruit:** I discovered that I could open a container of blue cheese crumbles without making any noise, and the aroma was unappealing to Sadie. These crumbles and fresh fruit, particularly apples, make a decent dessert.

- **Ice Cream:** Yep, thanks to Sadie's good doc, ice cream appeared in my life once again. However, after that initial splurge with the New York Super Fudge Chunk, I discovered some great low-calorie ice-cream bars located right near the Frosty Paws in the supermarket freezer. Contentment arrived at last: Sadie and her Frosty Paws—me and my frozen fudge bars (see shopping list, page 221).

- **Jell-O:** Despite Bill Cosby's testimonials, Jell-O still reigns as the favorite dessert of hospitals, jails, mental institutions and rehab centers. Of course, the situation in my home before Sadie's arrival and our new diet was much like any one of these establishments, but Jell-O has taken on a new exalted position on the food chain for me. It's quiet, has no smell, is sweet, and on top of all that, the sugar-free kind tastes no different than the regular kind and only has ten calories. You can even add a dollop of whipped cream for extra delight—it just can't be the kind in the spray can because of the noise it makes.

- **Ricotta Cheese:** Combined with different flavorings and a little sweetener, ricotta cheese makes a decent dessert that has no aroma and is quiet as well. Try blueberries or instant coffee, cocoa, lime juice, vanilla flavoring or any other imaginative substance you can think of.

The food part of the Dog Diet was established. I didn't concern myself too much with a lack of variety because I was eating in peace, Sadie was eating reasonably, and I'd gotten a lot thinner and a whole lot happier. However, I had an embarrassing incident on a rare day that I happened to go out to my favorite Indian buffet for lunch. If you love Indian food like I do, you know that part of its allure is the many fantastic aromas it emits. I found myself standing at the buffet unaware that I was actually sniffing the air. It had been such a long time since I had really smelled any great food aromas that I was lost in the moment, enjoying all the exquisite fragrances emanating from the various dishes. The friend I was with poked me in the back, making me aware of my strange behavior. Initially, I was chagrined, realizing she wasn't the only person who had noticed me sniffing the air. Seems everyone in the buffet line had frozen, plates in hand, as they stared at me. I recovered in a short time and laughed. I mean, after all, I couldn't have been more like Sadie. Only I didn't stick my head under the buffet table hood and sniff right at the source.

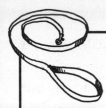

Dog Diet
DISCOVERIES

1. Consider the cost of losing weight! Your dog is the best deal out there.

2. Foods with tempting aromas can often be the worst food for a diet.

3. Foods that cause a dilemma with your dog are foods to avoid.

4. Cold food is a good choice. Your body has to burn more calories to warm it up, and you also won't eat as much.

5. Eating foods you can share with your dog makes mealtimes happier.

CHAPTER FIVE

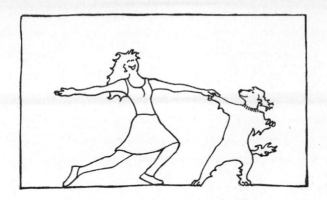

Revving Up Your Metabolism

(Letting the leash lead you)

*A*s spring turned into early summer, I found myself shaking off the final threads of my winter's despair. Sadie's quirks, which I first saw as irritating disruptions, were now part of my daily life. Now that I could sleep all night and wake up on my own, I was just generally well rested and therefore could function better (I actually couldn't remember eating dog food in a sleepy haze). Things do seem to go better when you're not launched into the day before dawn by shrill barking! I could even eat regular meals in peace now. Okay, maybe they weren't what the culinary world would call normal, but they worked for us.

The pounds were coming off without any organized effort on my part. I wasn't measuring anything, writing everything down, keeping track of each and every morsel of food or activity that comprised my day. I was lighter physically, and I was feeling lighter psychologically and emotionally. The many things that used to upset me now made me laugh. I wasn't lonely anymore either. Go figure!

It was a bright morning filled with sunshine. I was on my way to my office in quite a merry mood. Having peacefully consumed a breakfast of cottage cheese with mango-peach salsa and two cups of hazelnut coffee, I was enjoying not only the lovely day, but also my overall feeling of goodwill and good health. I was in high gear—and I knew it wasn't just the coffee.

After years of diet supplements, exercise and methods bordering on witchcraft to get my metabolism going, I felt I'd finally accomplished it. But how? What was "metabolism" anyway? I'd never really understood this invisible mechanism, which by all accounts held the secret to weight loss and control. Every diet had some scheme for increasing your metabolism, which in turn should result in weight loss. Like calorie counting, it was an integral and crucial component of almost all diets I had ever attempted. But I'm one of those skeptics who have to be able to see and touch something, and the only results I ever saw from too many calories or a slow metabolism were that my clothes didn't fit and my face looked puffy. How these intangible entities did this to me was often more puzzling than balancing my checkbook.

Webster's New World Dictionary defines metabolism as "the chemical and physical processes continuously going on in living organisms and cells, comprising those by which assimilated food is built up (anabolism) into protoplasm and those by which protoplasm is used and broken down (catabolism) into simpler substances or waste matter, with the release of energy for all vital processes." Huh?

Based on my own personal history I translated this to mean that most of my adult life, I engaged in extreme anabolism, adding lots of protoplasm to my body, which just hung around because I never seemed to get the catabolism part right. I consumed too much food, and my body was never able to use it all up, so it stored it as fat. The dictionary's definition made it sound like this metabolism thing was something beyond my control, which of course is not the case.

I'd tried diets that touted eating certain foods guaranteed to "put your metabolism into high gear." A week eating those foods left me exhausted, even if my only physical exertion each day was actually walking to the refrigerator to get them. Another fitness program advocated twenty minutes of a grueling routine on the treadmill *immediately* upon rising in the morning and *before* you were allowed to eat anything. Many were the mornings after those twenty-minute endurance sessions that I could barely pull myself up the basement steps. Rather than speeding up my metabolism, it just seemed to shut it down.

My worst attempts at fast-forwarding my metabolism had to be the countless supplements I swallowed that swore on their money-back guarantee that one of these capsules a day would do it. Anyone who's ever taken some form of these supposed miracle pills and lived to tell about it can confirm what happened to me. After ingesting some of these pills, I couldn't even hold a cup of coffee without shaking, let alone get it to my mouth without spilling it on my clothes. Once I was so nervous from one of these concoctions that I was afraid to leave my apartment. They made me talk too fast, sweat profusely and eat more than I would have without them.

Yep, those little devils made me overeat for two reasons. One, I thought if they were diluted in my stomach with food, the bad effects would wear off sooner. But my crazy thinking also made me believe that this food-burning furnace inside of me was now a raging inferno, and anything I ingested would quickly disappear in the flames. Wrong on both counts. I might be the only person alive that has actually gained weight while taking fat-burning metabolism-raising pills, but I doubt it.

What the dictionary didn't define, and what all those diet programs had not addressed, was "mental metabolism." Sure, Sadie had given my energy levels the equivalent of shock treatments with all the many daily demands of dog duties, but my new awareness went beyond that. In my experience, diets were all about deprivation, and that alone is a downer. And yes, Sadie had deprived me of food as well as sleep, but the lift she'd given to my mental metabolism to keep my body moving was fabulous.

Granted, Sadie had certainly gotten me more active, and most of the time not by choice or even willingly, but there was more to it than movement. It was also about mood. She approached every morning and each aspect of her life in such an exuberant manner, it was rubbing off on me. If Sadie is a typical dog, then dogs in general greet mornings differently than do humans. This difference could be the reason that, in the past, I'd been unable to get this metabolism thing going, which in turn would have jump-started my weight loss and perhaps ended many years of diet craziness. I decided to take a closer look at what Sadie did in the mornings. What I discovered was surprising. There certainly was more to metabolism than burning the excess calories I seemed destined to ingest, and I had unknowingly been learning it from my little dog. Starting with when she opened her eyes and ending when she went into her crate when I went to work, her actions and mood had changed mine, and all for the better.

Pay attention to your dog; see if you don't uncover actions and attitudes similar to Sadie's. Then see if your life won't be a whole lot better, not to mention your metabolism faster, if you adopt them for yourself.

Now that Sadie was sleeping with me, I was sleeping better. A lifelong insomniac, I had always tossed and turned during the night. My nights were interspersed with short periods of television, reading and, worst of all, eating. Because the food I ate at lunch had always made me tired, my justification for this nighttime grazing was that it would help me fall back to sleep. Now the only thing that awakened me during the night was a bark from Sadie if she detected a noise that might mean danger, or her occasional snoring.

When I woke up in the morning, I was no longer tired. Each morning, Sadie would greet me with the rapid thumping of her tail on the bed and scootch up from the bottom of the bed where she slept. The minute she detected that my eyes were open, I'd hear that high-speed tail hitting the mattress, and she'd jump on me and lick me fully awake. How could anyone possibly wake up in a bad mood or be reluctant to face the day with such an enthusiastic hello? I was laughing and moving quickly to avoid more jumping and licking as I got out of bed.

This was the beginning of my metabolic charge each day, and I realized I was probably burning more calories before I even got to the kitchen than I might have used during an entire day of lying on the couch that miserable winter.

A happy mood just pepped me up, got me going and made me feel that my day, even my existence, had a purpose. I didn't want to turn over and avoid the day anymore. I don't know if there's any scientific data to support my theory that waking up happy gives your metabolism a boost, but I choose to believe it. New morning rituals evolved, which I think are parts of a supercharged morning metabolism. These got my mornings off to a great start and kept me moving all day as well. Here are some new routines to add to your morning that will get you moving—mentally and physically.

1. Splash some cold water on your face . . . not ice-cube cold, just enough to feel refreshed. Wash your face with a mint scrub such as Benefit's Fantasy Mint Wash.

2. Stretch with your dog. Sadie has an elaborate morning

stretching ritual. The human version of it goes something like this: Lie facedown on the floor with your arms outstretched. Push your hands and feet forward as far as you can, elongating your body as much as possible. Bring your hands back to your hips, and lift your upper body up, arching your back and neck backward. Keeping your back arched, let your head hang down as you relax your neck muscles. Shake your head . . . pretend you have floppy ears that you're swinging around. Do this three times. Bring your body into a curled position, knees drawn to your chest, arms hugging the tight ball your body is now in. Stand up slowly. At this point Sadie would just wriggle in delight. Put your arms straight out to your sides, parallel to the floor, and twist from side to side as you loosen your waist muscles. Then I always pat my chest and Sadie jumps up, and I catch her for a morning hug.

3. Make your bed before going for coffee.

4. Get dressed before going downstairs or to the kitchen.

5. Engage in a few rounds of tug-of-war with your dog or get down on the floor and have a little wrestling match. According to a popular Web site, (*www.caloriesperhour.com*) you can burn 97 calories in twenty minutes of vigorous play with your dog.

6. Turn on some music to keep you moving. Research has shown that listening to feel-good music taps into that same feel-good center of your brain that eating your favorite foods does.

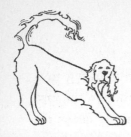

7. Lift your dog up three times to face level. (Unless she weighs 100 lbs!)
8. Hang up any clothes thrown on the floor or chair from the night before.
9. Race your dog to the kitchen.

Sound silly? Think of it as your first calorie deficit deposit for the day. Each of these activities is stimulating, accomplishes a task or serves some purpose, and puts you on the road back into those special jeans!

Sniffing the New Day

Sadie's routine soon didn't require that I accompany her out for her initial morning pee. I'd open the back door, and she'd run into the yard, but the first thing she always did was stop and sniff the air. She'd stand in the middle of the patio, head tilted back, just taking small whiffs of the air.

In those early days with Sadie, I had also done a lot of sniffing—to see if she had sneaked off to a corner of the house for a bathroom break when I was unaware. I'd enter each room, nose in ultraperceptive mode, and I'd sniff out all the corners and under all the furniture. To her credit it only happened once, and I sprayed the elixir that had been suggested to me by another dog parent, and Sadie never did it again. I also had honed my olfactory sense to a science during the development of the food part of the Dog Diet, but aside from actually stopping and smelling some roses, I hadn't made a practice of sniffing the air first thing every morning.

I tried this and found it invigorating. The fresh morning air is enticing and energizing. When I stood that first time in the yard with Sadie and sniffed the morning air, I could faintly detect the smell of my roses, the evergreens, the lingering smell of the citronella candles from the night before, my coffee drifting out from the kitchen and the soft odor of Sadie's piña colada shampoo on her fur as the morning sun warmed her. Soon Sadie would scamper to the back of the yard and take a pee, and together we'd run back into the house—me to my coffee, Sadie to her water bowl.

The new day had a fresh smell, and I soon realized that scent could be an important part of motivating my metabolism. Essential oils have long been touted as cures for numerous ailments and conditions. Lavender is said to promote restful sleep. Ylang-ylang is relaxing, while citrus scents are energizing. (Some of my favorite scented products are listed under "Necessary Luxuries and Scents for Mealtime Moments and More" on page 229.)

Even perfume can play a role in your metabolism rate. Certain perfumes contain pheromones, which are supposed to attract the opposite sex. These leave you feeling lustful, which, granted, is sometimes a great feeling, but first thing in the morning, when you need to get your metabolism revved up, you don't want to be feeling languid and slow-moving. Other perfumes have a fresh and clean fragrance that just make you feel good about yourself and are invigorating. Choose one of these for a supercharged day. A fresh, clean-smelling perfume will do wonders for making your mental metabolism skip right along at a steady pace; once your mental metabolism is in gear, your body will follow. Why someone hasn't created a perfume called "Morning" is beyond me.

Here's how you can incorporate scent into your morning to energize your metabolism and your spirit:

1. Start the night before. Spray a citrus scent on your bedside lamp before going to bed. In the morning when you turn it on, the heat from the bulb will infuse the scent into the air, sending a feeling of energy right into your senses.
2. Set your coffeemaker to start your coffee before you go to bed. Flavored coffee is the best for this. My favorite is hazelnut. Before you even open your eyes, the scent of the coffee comes wafting up the stairs . . . you might even wake up *before* your dog!
3. Try to keep some fresh flowers in your kitchen. Freesia are inexpensive and have a wonderful fragrance.
4. Eat some citrus. Fresh oranges and grapefruit are wonderful choices to start your day with, and the smell is revitalizing. These are foods that your dog will not beg you for either!
5. Use a stimulating shower gel or body scrub. Citrus, rosemary, chocolate, coffee and ginger are all great scents to get you moving.
6. Spray your sheets with scented linen spray. These sprays come in many different lovely, light scents that make falling asleep and waking up quite pleasant.
7. Put some potpourri in your car's ashtray.

8. Use a fruit- or mint-flavored lip gloss.
9. Keep some scented candles on hand at home and at work if possible.
10. On your morning walks, take time to notice the fresh scents of the morning such as flowers, breakfast cooking smells and freshly cut grass.

Scent also evokes pleasant memories from past associations. We all have fond recollections associated with certain scents. When I was clerking for a firm during law school, I went to an insurance company for depositions where they baked fresh bread daily. They said it made the employees relaxed and productive at the same time. It only made me want more than one piece slathered with a generous amount of real butter. I was lucky I was only there for two days.

Surrounding yourself with scents that have pleasant associations is a boost for your mood and will be reflected in your movements. When your mind is humming along with happy thoughts, your body can't help but skip right along. Now that the foods you're eating are mostly odorless, you need to use other methods to keep your sense of smell in tip-top shape.

A word of caution, however, concerning food-scented candles. I thought they would serve two purposes: first, they would satisfy my deprived sense of smell, as my meals no longer sent enticing odors throughout the house, and second, they would function as a substitute for the foods I was unable to eat. I really thought these delightful imitations for such longed-for items as chocolate cake, gingerbread, apple pie and lemon meringue pie would be just the ticket. There are even candles that are scented like wine, merlot and chardonnay to be precise. Their scents are unbelievably realistic, and they only make you want the real thing even more, so forget it.

I started with a cake-infused candle in the entranceway of my house. Sadie and I returned from our walk to the delightful smell of a baking cake. Immediately her nose went into action as did mine. She ran into the kitchen, searching in vain for the source of this perceived treat. She started barking and stood up to sniff the top of the kitchen island as she looked at me for help. This was unnerving for me too. I ended up eating all the leftover chocolate in the refrigerator, and Sadie searched the entire first floor of the house for the nonexistent cake. This was the end of my experimentation with food-scented candles.

Morning Walkies

Remember Barbara Woodhouse, the English dog trainer who popularized the phrase "walkies"? You could hear the energy in her lilting voice as she encouraged the dog at the end of the leash to get off to a brisk and lively walk, and the dog took off to the command of "walkies." I remembered this as I watched Sadie begin her walk every morning.

Sadie never walked out the front door slowly. While she'd go out the back door for her initial morning pee in a slow, contemplative manner, it was not so with the front door. Going out the front meant we were going to greet the world outside. With all the enthusiasm she could generate, she'd jerk me out the door and off the porch right along with her. This walk was full of promising discoveries, and the sooner we got going, the better.

Thanks to waking up in a good mood, not to mention a strong cup of aromatic coffee, I was ready to greet the day along with her. So many times in the past, I'd just run out my door for a quick walk whose only purpose was to try to burn a few measly calories and get that mystical metabolism moving up a notch or two. Now, instead of enduring a walk I believed mandatory to lose weight, I was enjoying it, and I was benefiting more from it. Not only was I down fifteen pounds, I had not agonized over each and every pound and had not so much as consulted one diet missive. Nor had I paced myself on any of these walks with Sadie, or worn a heart monitor, or counted the minutes until I got home.

While I didn't have unlimited time to devote to this walk before work, I made time for it by getting up earlier. You'd be surprised how much you can get done if you wake up in a good mood and as little as a half hour before your normal time.

As time went on, we adopted certain things in these walks that I realized were aiding in my weight loss and became part of the Dog Diet regimen. Here are some ideas that we used that you can incorporate in your morning walk with your dog.

1. Take your walk each morning at a regular time. This doesn't mean to the exact second where you put undue stress on yourself in the morning. Just make it part of your morning

routine. The walk is kind of like having coffee: you want it and it makes you feel good—but the walk is good for your dog as well.

2. Have a time parameter for the walk. If you can spare a half hour, great. If you have more time, better, but if you only have twenty minutes, so be it.

3. Don't let the weather discourage you. Rain or shine, warm or cold, this is part of your morning ritual. Sure, most of us want to roll over on rainy days and sleep a little longer, but people only burn 57 calories per hour sleeping. Compare this to burning 174 calories in sixty minutes of walking your dog, and your choice is clear.

4. Eat a small portion of protein before your walk. A hard-boiled egg is great because both you and your dog can have one. It will keep you from being famished when you return to the kitchen, and some diet specialists out there swear that you burn more calories if you eat a small amount of protein prior to exercising.

5. If you don't feel good, go for the walk anyway. Don't get lazy and just turn your dog out into the backyard for her bathroom break. Take it slower, don't go as far, but do go. Keep up the routine, and more than likely, you'll feel better when you get back from the walk. Remember, sometimes getting up is half the battle!

6. Let your dog set the pace. Sadie always wants to run short lengths and then walk slower. She repeats this throughout our walk several times. It turns out that interval training (what you pay the trainers big bucks to teach you) is excellent for giving

your metabolism a nudge. Bursts of high-intensity activity are a surefire way to boost your metabolism. Add a thirty-second sprint every five minutes of your walk, or if you only have ten minutes, add a thirty-second speed-up every three minutes. For some reason we probably wouldn't understand or would forget, this speeds up the burning of fat more than consistent, paced aerobic exercise.

7. If one side of the street where you take your walk is sunny and the other shady, stick to the sunny side. Sunshine is good for you despite the skin cancer warnings. Unless you're walking naked at the speed of a tortoise, you're just fine facing the morning sun. I wear a ball cap and sunglasses in the morning. Of course, my other reason for donning these items is that I'm pretty scary looking first thing in the morning, and while Sadie is happy to see me in any state, my neighbors might not be! But seriously, the sunshine is cheerful, helps you get your vitamin D, and yet another diet guru says that sunlight helps curb our appetites, thus controlling intake of calories. (Why, then, did I order all those margaritas while on the beach?)

8. Observe your surroundings as you walk. Take a moment to explore things that catch your dog's interest. These little detours add distance to your walk, hence increasing calorie burning. Letting the leash lead you—following your dog's lead—is the only plan you need.

9. Vary your route. If one day you go *down* the street, go *up* the street the next day. Try to do at least a mile on each walk, even at noon. It doesn't take that long, and you won't get bored.

10. If there's a set of stairs on your route, try carrying your dog up
    them. I know this won't work if your dog is a Great Pyrenees, but
    an average-size dog is fine for this. Carrying a sixteen- to twenty-
    four-pound dog up stairs for three minutes burns an extra 17
    calories. This might not seem like much, but it all adds up.

We also walked at noon when I came home for lunch and again
in the evening. Our evening walks were much longer and more
social as the boulevard where we walk is where every dog and their
mom or dad also walks in the evening. Don't be discouraged if you
can't go home for lunch and take a walk with your dog. Walk from
your job to pick up your lunch, imagining you are walking your
dog, and if you have one of those "eat at your desk jobs," just take
a mental walk—it will still rev up your metabolism.

On very late winter afternoons or early evenings, when it's really
cold, wet, dark and bone-chilling, I opt for the treadmill after a quick
dash out for Sadie's relief trip. The first time I used the treadmill,
Sadie was overly curious. She kept coming nearer, and I kept telling
her to get back. Finally, she just hopped on before I could grab her,
and just as swiftly, she was catapulted off the belt and into the wall.
Talk about your adrenaline rising and in turn your metabolism!

I turned to look at her when she jumped on, and as she went flying off, I too lost my balance, fell into the cord holding the emergency shut-off key, which pulled it out and abruptly stopped the
treadmill, and I fell off as well. From then on she stayed away from
the treadmill, and it had to be an extremely nasty day outside for
me to opt for indoor exercise.

Keep Busy

I have nothing against relaxing. After all, I spent an entire winter as close to a state of inertia as I believe a human being can. But inactivity does nothing to stoke your internal calorie-burning furnace. With a dog, you rarely have the time to sit, let alone relax: feeding, bathing, playing and walking your dog are all activities that of course burn calories. But puppies create many situations that require reparative action on your part, and instead of getting frustrated with my dog, I learned to appreciate the opportunities that I hadn't had before to burn all those extra calories.

I mean, why sit and file your nails if you can be gathering up half-chewed rawhide pieces from all over the house or trying to get the bite marks off your miniblinds? Here are some other situations where your dog makes you take action and helps forgo those states of inertia—things that will get you moving and push your metabolism to a higher level. These seemingly resting activities take on a new level when a dog comes into the picture. No longer are you able to do just one thing; nope, dogs are the original multitaskers!

1. **Reading Magazines:** Sadie always felt left out when I tried to read anything. She'd come up on the couch and try to get between me and the magazine, with toys and other disturbances. Don't ignore this! Comply with your dog's every request because it's in your best interest! If she jumps up on the couch, stand up and lift her down. If she brings you the ball, throw it to her between reading sentences. All of these little interruptions are opportunities to expend more calories.

2. **Watching Television:** Sadie watched Animal Planet all day while I was at work, so she had no tolerance for my wanting to sit in front of the TV. I discovered that I could watch television out of the corner of my eye if I lay on the floor and played with her. I'd absentmindedly throw Mr. Cheeseburger into the hall endlessly, just to get the gist of the evening world news. Watching television as you lie on the couch quietly burns only 58 calories in an entire hour, while just moderate play activity with your dog uses up 77 calories in only twenty minutes. And if you kick it up a notch to a vigorous level, which would include some tug-of-war and a few lifts up in the air along with wrestling, you'll burn almost 100 calories in those twenty minutes!

3. **Eating:** I've already detailed the many struggles involved in eating; however, while ingesting your calories, you can also be increasing how quickly you use them up. I found it easier to avoid Sadie's begging by standing up at my kitchen island and eating. Turns out preparing your food at home instead of cruising through the drive-through of the nearest fast-food restaurant will knock off 48 calories in twenty minutes, and eating it standing up will burn 12 calories in six minutes. Okay, that's probably not even one bite's worth of food, but every little bit helps. And it depends on what you're eating. Think about it, if you're just having a green salad and take your time eating it, you might even end up with a calorie deficit!

4. **Tearing Up the Garden:** One of the questions the adoption

counselor at PetSmart asked me was if I had a fenced-in yard where the dog could play. Sure I did. I have a lovely, little secret-garden oasis with an eight-foot privacy fence. Compared to what Sadie had been used to at the shelter, I assured the lady this backyard would be heavenly. I couldn't have been more wrong. Then again, in the beginning, I had been pretty much off track with everything concerning dog parenting. I did all I could to get Sadie to appreciate this little garden sanctuary, but she only tolerated it when I was out there with her. The times I'd leave her alone, she panicked, barked and dug up my garden. The work involved in replacing everything was tiresome, but it did have its upside. Gardening is a good activity for burning calories. In fifteen minutes of digging, I used up 73 calories, 13 more than the ice-cream fudge bar I ate when I discovered my lemongrass plant had disappeared. And when the destruction was greater and I had to replant the garden all over again, I kissed off 261 calories in just one hour!

5. **Cleaning:** My house was no longer a showcase for any of the numerous cleaning products I'd once used with abandon. But I did try to keep up some semblance of order, and Sadie's mishaps and endless hair loss kept me busy. I even had to purchase a new vacuum cleaner, which I used almost daily. This, too, is not a bad deal, because cleaning the house gives you even more opportunities to move the metabolism along faster. In a normal household, vacuuming for only fifteen minutes will burn up 51 calories. In one

where a dog lives, it's harder, because Sadie, as I discovered was true of most dogs, was afraid of the sweeper. The maneuvers I had to go through to get the floor swept were intricate and time-consuming, and I am convinced must have at least doubled my calorie expenditure. And when I finally got to put the monster sweeper away, I wasn't done. Hair control only began with vacuuming. Then I had to mop. I always mopped my floor on my hands and knees, which used up an additional 102 calories in thirty minutes. By the time I'd completed my feeble attempts to eradicate the dog hair polluting my house, I was famished, but at least I'd earned the right to indulge in a few extra calories. I'd burned them up *before* I even ate them!

6. **Changing the Sheets:** The morning I opened my eyes and saw nothing but dog hair on my pillowcase was frightening. *How could this be happening?* I thought. *Surely this dog will soon look like a Mexican hairless, and the infinite task of capturing all this hair will be over.* I started running a sticky lint remover over her before bed, which cut down on the hairy pillows. I still had to change my sheets more often, which is also a good calorie-burning activity. You erase 48 calories in twenty minutes of changing linen. If you think that changing the bed doesn't take that long and isn't that challenging, you've not tried doing it with a dog under your feet.

7. **Maintaining the Car:** I had not expected the hair war to carry over to my car, but it did. Sadie was an excellent driving companion, even though she hated waiting alone while I

ran into a store. I soon realized that no matter how nice my car appeared inside when we left the house, it never returned that way. To ease her anxiety at my ten-minute or less absences, she'd lick every window in the car, hop from the front seat to the back, spreading yet more dog hair in places it didn't belong and, for reasons unknown, slobbered all over the steering wheel. I could never offer anyone a ride after Sadie had accompanied me somewhere. I soon was cleaning the car about three times a week. Even after I started putting a cover on Sadie's seat, the windows and floors still needed attention. Not one to do a halfway job, I'd also wash the exterior, burning up a hefty 87 calories in thirty minutes.

8. **Snacking:** Sadie wanted treats all the time and would sit expectantly by the drawer in the kitchen where I kept them. Snacking on the right things is good for losing weight. Make a habit of taking breaks from whatever you're doing and have a snack between meals right along with your dog. Sadie loves little peanut butter treats, and I'll have a piece of celery with peanut butter. Or she will indulge in a dog cookie, and I'll have a piece of fruit, and sometimes we both just have some cottage cheese. Frequent eating keeps your metabolism running along at a faster pace all day. Our last snack was an hour before bedtime. Sadie had a Frosty Paws, and I'd have some cottage cheese with fruit or salsa.

9. **Drinking Water:** Dogs drink a *lot* of water. I'd refill Sadie's water bowl many times during the day, and when I came home for lunch or after work, the first thing she did when I

let her out of her pennie was drink an entire bowl of water. I always knew that drinking water was good for you, but we get busy and forget, so every time I'd hear Sadie noisily lapping up water in the kitchen, I'd get a glass of water for me too. Water is refreshing, is a good appetite suppressant and steps up your metabolism as well. Who knew? But a German study found that when you drink 17 ounces of water, within twenty minutes your metabolic rate shoots up by about 30 percent! Factor in that Sadie likes her water with ice cubes, which results in extra work for me, and of course, extra calories burned up by me. The body uses extra calories just to warm up ice water, which makes it a clear choice above room temperature water.

10. **Play:** Take the time to play with your dog. Sure, I fit playtime in with other activities, but taking at least a half hour just to play with Sadie was a surefire way to get my metabolism moving. Inventing silly games, chasing her, letting her chase me, throwing balls, jumping over things in the backyard, tug-of-war and any other conceivable physical activity with her many toys made playtime a fun time for both of us. In *Ageless Body, Timeless Mind,* Deepak Chopra says that each adult person should do one thing every day that they remember as pleasant from childhood. This can be as simple as eating an ice-cream cone or riding a swing. With Sadie it was easy to escape to a childish pleasure with complete abandon. I did answer the phone, rather out of breath, during one of these play sessions. When the puzzled caller asked

what I was doing, I didn't think before answering, "Chasing squirrels." The silence on the other end of the phone was deafening. We just barked and hung up.

As you see, in addition to walking, it's possible to burn a large number of calories just in the activities you must do with your dog and the many tasks she creates for you to do around the house. Even giving her a bath supposedly burns 68 calories in twenty minutes, but I think it has to be at least three times that number. By the time I'd chase her down, brush her teeth, get her down to the basement and place her in the paint sink where she got her bath, apply the shampoo, scrub her down, dry her off, untangle her ears and change my wet clothes, I was exhausted. Then I had to wash all the towels we used, dry them and fold them. One semi-wet dog would then run up the basement stairs, and I would follow, dragging my feet. At this point, my metabolism was running so fast it was wearing me out.

There was no doubt my activity level had increased dramatically, and it certainly had to be playing a significant role in my weight loss. The secret was that most of these activities were done without a conscious effort on my part at all. They were just part of my routine. The morning walks have become as normal as drinking a cup of coffee.

Metabolism, that mythical, invisible key to weight loss, can become your friend instead of an unsolved mystery that serves as an excuse for your excess weight. Follow your dog's lead whether she's tugging you along as you hold her leash or creating opportunities for you to get moving in other ways.

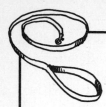

Dog Diet
DISCOVERIES

1. Metabolism is not a mystery and good moods get it moving!

2. Greet the morning like your dog—with a "bring on the day" attitude!

3. Use invigorating scents to boost your mental metabolism.

4. Duties of dog care aren't burdens—they're calorie consumers!

5. When your mind is humming happy thoughts, your body will skip along.

CHAPTER SIX

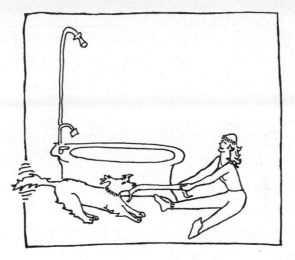

Dogercise

(Workouts when you least expect them)

Despite the myriad of failures that made up my dieting history, I'd been dragged into an eating plan that was working. Of course, it was structured around being able to eat anything at all, not everything in sight as had been my lifelong habit. I also had a new mental attitude that kept me going each day in a cheerful mode. Sadie had succeeded in ending my indulgent food practices and banished the gloom that had controlled my winter slump.

Now it was time to confront that second component of all diet programs, exercise. I, for one, have always associated the word "endure" with the word exercise. I can't say I'd ever found a program of exercise that I really enjoyed. However, all the experts— those I read and those I employed and paid dearly—said that in order to be successful with a program of physical activity, you had to like it. How could this be? I've already told you about the personal trainers I had and the ridiculous rigid parameters they squeezed my life into while in their custody. During these torturous periods, they may have gotten my body squeezed into a size or two smaller, but it never lasted, and there certainly wasn't any part of it that was even close to pleasant.

The TV infomercials for exercise equipment must all certainly be elaborate hoaxes. You know—those smiling slim people who seem to have the time of their lives while rocking their abs into cement-like consistency or swinging their legs wildly on some contraption named after a wild animal. There's no way they can be expressing true delight at such activities. I should know, because I've tried them all and purchased at least half of them. Take a tour through my house, and you'll see what I mean. From a complete set of free weights with a bench, to rubber bands of various sizes and elasticity, to my all-time favorite flop, the Thigh Master, I have them all. My basement looks like a gym's rummage sale, and the truth is, I got a lot of those discarded fitness dream-machines from other people who had also failed miserably at accomplishing anything at all with them.

The only thing I didn't fall for was that electronic contraption you strapped on, did absolutely nothing and still lost weight. This device supposedly shoots electrical currents through the stored fat in your body and jars it loose. The commercials for it were so convincing that I thought I might actually stand a chance of having a decent time while using it. People were even eating pizza while wearing this device and losing weight to boot! The only reason I was able to resist buying this miracle pound zapper was because I asked my doctor about it. (My doctor had a lot in common with me and was quite understanding of all my weight-loss debacles. He, too, always had a few pounds he wanted to shed and, in general, was a sympathetic ear to my travails in this department. He often cheated on his health-conscious wife when she was out of town—with hot dogs and Oreo cookies.) Had he even slightly indicated a remote chance of success with this electrical fat eliminator, I would've had one FedExed to me immediately.

There had been periods of time when I'd spend the entire evening walking around my house with ankle weights on, in the mistaken belief that they were somehow erasing the damage wrought on my body by the chicken and dumplings or hot roast beef sandwich I'd consumed. I'd even lie on the couch and watch television with them on in hopes of losing a few measly ounces. My hit-and-miss method of using these contraptions might possibly have something to do with why they never worked, but I doubt it.

I used my treadmill the most because I could watch television while running on it. I even became obsessed with it while following a regimen that required aerobic exercise immediately after every meal. I soon saw why this method could work. I'd get so sick to my stomach from the vigorous exertion right after eating that I soon began eating very little at mealtime. The program, however, said nothing about exercising after snacking, so I just began eating large snacks. While breakfast might consist of a cup of coffee and a piece of fruit, followed by twenty minutes on the treadmill, any progress was negated by the sandwich or two I'd eat at my desk midmorning. Needless to say, this program did not last very long.

Once, I religiously followed a popular plan to transform my body, and it worked to a certain degree. However, it was so strenuous and demanded not only a lot of time, but six meals a day, which in turn necessitated specialized grocery shopping and massive opportunities for cheating. You were allowed one day a week where you could eat whatever you wanted. I think the idea behind this was that you wouldn't always crave the things that would cause you to regain the weight you had worked so hard to lose. Ha! If they only knew. The feelings of deprivation were so huge that I ate more in that one day than I did the entire week while following the guidelines of the program. I'd feel so guilty after my one-day food orgy, that I starved myself the rest of the week to make up for it. After twelve weeks, it simply wore me out, and no matter how thin and spectacular I could envision myself looking down the road, I couldn't keep it up.

Keeping track of all the eating was hard enough, but the exercises were exhausting. Each exercise required a progressively heavier set of free weights, which, in turn, demanded even more assistance from a personal trainer. There were mornings I could barely drive home from the gym and days when I ached so much I could hardly move. There was no way this system was ever going to evolve into even the most meager form of enjoyment.

I joined a gym for more than one reason. I thought maybe group participation would hasten my weight-loss endeavors, and had read that gyms were great places to meet men. Whoever said the gym was replacing the bar as the new social meeting ground hasn't been to the bars I've been to. The bars I frequented only involved movement from one bar stool to another depending on where the good-looking guys were, signaling to get the bartender's attention and bending your elbow. There was no sweating (okay, maybe a time or two a sweat did break out from nerves), but there was no flexing of muscles, and I was much better at matching mental muscles with my snappy repartees than any flexing I'd done at the gym. And I actually met an interesting guy or two at these watering holes who were good for at least a few decent dinners. But the only ones I met at the gym were the ones that scared me with their bulk and made me shy away from using any machines in their vicinity. Bars and gyms, and the men who frequent them, have little in common.

My experiences in the organized fitness classes were just as futile as my attempts to meet men there. Not only were the classes not fun, they were downright embarrassing. At least in the privacy of my own home I could pop in a video and exercise without witnesses. After all, I could always stop the tape, rewind it and start again. Not that I ever actually did that; more often than not, I'd cruise to the kitchen for a snack and return to the television in time to get in on the finale. I don't think I ever watched one to the end. While my video library would lead you to believe I could operate a myriad of complex home fitness machines, sweat to the oldies or kickbox with zeal, my physical condition told the real story: These tapes rarely made it out of their cases into the VCR.

In a regimented gym class you can't just leave the room for a candy bar or stand idle while everyone follows the instructor. Well, actually you can if you're in the very back corner of the room, but you have to get to the class very early to get this spot, and you can't leave it for a second or someone will take it. The simplest aerobic moves seemed monumental to me. I was never in sync with the class, and I was constantly out of breath. Truth is, I left these sessions feeling like the most out-of-shape person in the universe. None of the camaraderie that group participation is supposed to foster had the slightest effect on me. I made no friends and engaged in no friendly competition. After the class, I just slinked out the door as quickly as possible, most often taking a detour to the McDonald's drive-through to soothe my shattered nerves. Try I did, though, from Jazzercise, to step classes and even to spinning. I gave them all my best shot, but only made the tiniest gains in fitness or weight loss.

Clothes were another reason I hated group exercise endeavors. At home you can wear anything or nothing at all, if you can stand the sight of yourself. But at the gym, there are always women who are in terrific shape and don't hide it under a large bulky T-shirt either. While they would look stunning in tight-fitting spandex, I'd show up in my sweatpants and misshapen T-shirt from some long ago vacation. I could never get the headband thing right. It would end up around my neck, pausing just long enough over my eyes to totally mess up any progress I was making at keeping in step. I felt like a whale out of water.

And so it went, one exercise program after another, and all the equipment that went along with them as well, discarded like failed experiments. In all my exhaustive efforts, the only thing I found that I could stretch the truth enough to say was maybe a little bit enjoyable was the treadmill. That is until Sadie came to live with me and I discovered "Dogercise." Each morning, Sadie came tumbling out of bed, energizing my spirit and taking me on a journey that evolved into exercise that was finally enjoyable, and, most of the time, I didn't even know I was doing it. Without any special equipment except my little shelter dog, no membership fees, no special clothes and no rigid rules, I was finally able to downsize myself when I entered the world of Dogercise.

As I've described, the extensive walking I was now doing with Sadie certainly gave a charge to my metabolism and my mood, but I felt I needed more. Sadie found it impossible to leave me alone with my feeble attempts at weight lifting and other attempts to get in shape. When I'd lie on the floor to do crunches, she'd bring toys over and drop them on my stomach. When I tried to use the contraption with the pulleys that you pulled yourself around on in a million different angles, she'd bite the ropes. Even attempting simple calf raises on the steps was impossible, as she'd bite my shoelaces.

One day, while getting her food out of the container on the back porch, I realized my movement was very similar to the squats I'd learned to do, which, in theory, were to tighten the back of my thighs. When I'd tried these in the basement with weights in each hand, I couldn't do them because Sadie would get underneath me, and I would've had to sit on her to finish the exercise. But *hold the puppy chow*—I could do these things as long as she was a part of them! And getting Sadie's food out of its container on the back porch was only the beginning!

I soon realized that almost every activity I did with Sadie was very similar to the standard exercises I'd spent years trying not to do. I'd actually been working out just through the necessary tasks of caring for her. It wasn't only about eating after all; in addition to the walks, I'd been exercising all along. I'd been Dogercising!

Through trial and error, I was soon able to adapt almost every task with Sadie into an exercise of some sort. No, they would not pass the rigid standards of trainers, and most likely would not be up to snuff with any fitness formulas. But they were fun and they were working. These are all very simple exercises. Finally, I'd found an enjoyable form of exercise. I knew I could do these for the rest of my life because most of the time I was putting no organized effort into them, they were just part of my day. Suddenly, sit-ups were a laughable matter with a small dog sitting on my stomach! No more embarrassment at my miserable performances in exercise classes. No more videotapes or wasting money on gadgets that I'd never be able to use. You can do these too with your dog, and both of you will have fun while getting fit.

The exercises I developed with Sadie are just guidelines. Depending on your dog's size and your imagination, everything is possible. The only rule for Dogercise is that it should be fun for both of you. Dogs are not lazy, and they can inspire us to shed our lethargic tendencies. You'll find more ways to burn calories

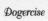

with your dog than you will possibly have time for if you just follow her lead. (Literally!)

Mealtime Squats

These were the first discovery in the development of Dogercise. It's very simple. I keep Sadie's food in an upright plastic container on the back porch. I stand in front of it, holding her bowl in one hand with my legs slightly apart and my feet turned out. I lower my body to the floor until my thighs are parallel with the floor. I then open the container and slowly rise back up. I repeat this and take the scoop out of the container on the second squat. On each successive squat, I get a small amount of food out of the container with the scoop and place it in her bowl. Not only does this give your thighs a workout, it helps develop balance, because your dog will be in the way. You'll have to dodge out of her way so you don't spill the food in the bowl while you're doing this exercise . . . ever hear of such a good combination for balance and toning?! It will keep her guessing how much food she's getting as well.

Breakfast Biceps

Sadie liked to eat her dry dog food mixed with canned dog food. I began playing a game with her as I used the cans to tone my biceps. They simply take the place of barbells. Stand in the kitchen with a can in each hand. Lower them to your side slowly and then raise them back to your shoulders. She could never figure out what I was doing exactly, but it looked like fun, so she'd jump at the cans and run around the kitchen island. I'd do three sets of fifteen repetitions.

A good variation of this exercise that is effective in reaching the inner part of the bicep area is to keep your elbows tight against your rib cage while turning your arms upward so your palms are facing the ceiling. Keep your elbows as tight to your sides as possible, then raise your prearms and lower them slowly. I did these slowly because I would tease Sadie with the cans, and it was fun to see her efforts to try to take them away from me. Sure, it made the exercises more difficult, but it was also more challenging.

You can use the cans for shoulder exercises as well. Hold your arms straight out with a can in each hand. Slowly lower your arms to your sides, and then back up parallel to the floor.

You can also do shoulder raises with them. Just hold the cans at shoulder level and then push your arms straight up as far as you can. Lower them slowly again to shoulder level.

Leash Triceps

A great number of women, including me, are most concerned with the triceps, or the back of the arm. How many of us have looked longingly at sleeveless dresses or have dreaded the arrival of summer because we are ashamed of the lack of shape our arms have? I've literally suffered through meetings and dinners refusing to take my jacket off for this very reason. (I tried over and over to learn how to use a fat caliper because this was one of the areas the trainers always took a measurement from. Turns out, if your dog is able to bite the extra fat on the back of your arm, it's time to tone them up!)

Right before her walk Sadie liked to play a crazy game with her leash. I felt it stretching these arm muscles and thus developed the "leash triceps." Attach the leash to your dog. With your arm straight down at your side, allow her to pull your arm backward as you hold the leash. As you gently pull the leash with her on the end of it back to your side, she will pull backward. This tension gives your triceps a great workout.

Walking Arm Toning

During your walk, keep your dog on the side away from the road both going and returning. This way each arm gets a good workout from holding the leash for half of the walk. Alternately keep your arm muscles taut and then release them. If your dog is like mine, and is wild with joy at just being outside even on a leash, your arms will get a good workout just keeping her under control. Her little bursts of energy along the way are good for your arms, and as she pulls you forward, you can gently bring her back to your side.

Bath Time Buffing

I believe I use every major muscle in my body just giving Sadie a bath. First I have to catch her, which can take fifteen minutes or more and involves more than one set of stairs. After she's captured, I have to lift her into the paint sink where she gets her bath. Now, when she was eight pounds this was no problem; however, as she grew, it became quite an effort. These baths always have to be performed quickly because I never know when she will bolt from the sink, and the last thing I need is a wet, soapy dog running all over the house.

Scrub your dog vigorously and do use a nicely scented special dog shampoo! (Rain forest and piña colada are our favorites.) Try to dry as much of her as possible while she is in the sink, because the real workout begins when she hits the floor and begins the mad after-bath dash. The actual drying process will be strenuous as you grab, lunge, pull and hold your dog in an attempt to get her dry. Give special attention and be gentle with her ears. My vet said it was important to keep dog's ears dry, but it also gives you a chance to catch your breath. Of course, it goes without saying that you both deserve a snack for a reward after this ordeal!

Tug-of-War

Sadie and I had tug-of-war with anything that she would pretend to give me and then abruptly change her mind and hang on to. From her tennis balls to my socks, anything was fair game in her give-and-keep schemes. Her favorite seemed to be the towel I attempted to dry her with after her bath. I'd be totally exhausted sitting on the floor; she'd grab one end of the towel and pull it from me. This works much like a rowing machine at the gym, but it's a lot livelier with a dog yanking on the towel. I sit on the floor with my legs stretched out in front of me holding one end of the towel. With Sadie holding on to the other end, I gently pull her toward me. This works your back, stomach and arm muscles. It is also a good stretch if you let your dog back up with the towel (or other object) while you continue to sit on the floor and bend forward, bringing your body as close to your legs as possible.

Dog Pull-Ups

This is a great back exercise and often follows the bath. The pull-up is an entertaining game with your dog. It starts out much like a tug-of-war, but goes a step further. Using a towel, allow your dog to grab on to one end of it. Pull her and the towel toward you while standing and continue to raise your hands to just under your chin as she hangs on to her end. Sadie considers this a real challenge, and I get worn out with it long before she ever wants to quit.

Dog Curls

Sadie loves to be cuddled and touched, and this exercise is one that she just loves. It happened accidentally as she jumped into my arms, and I lifted her close to my chest to make sure she didn't fall. I could feel the muscles in my arms working and repeated the movement much to her delight. Hold your dog firmly in your bent arms and bring her toward your chest. You will feel your bicep and tricep muscles working as you both lift and lower your arms and dog. On the last rep, you can lower her to the floor, giving your back a good stretch. Be prepared—she'll think this is just the beginning of a great game and jump all over you wanting more. The great thing about this is that you can do it anytime she comes begging for some attention—hugging your arms into sleek proportions!

Rubber Band Dog

I had purchased a kit of rubber band tubes for stretching and toning, but rarely used them. I took them on lots of business trips with me, but they always remained in the suitcase, and to my disappointment, I never saw the results promised on the television promos. Their claim to fitness perfection was resistance. I found that using Sadie in their place was a lot more effective and didn't require the extra equipment. It goes like this: Hook your dog to the leash and then loop the handle around your ankle. While standing up with your hand on the wall or a chair, slowly extend your leg straight out, and you will be floored (I hope not literally) by the resistance your dog will provide by pulling on the leash. Repeat this several times with each leg.

The rubber tubes were not a complete waste of money after all. Sadie loves to grab an end of one of them and pull it as far as she can stretch it. I get a good workout just trying to get the tubes back from her.

Puppy Push-Ups

This one is a lot of fun, and it doesn't take a great number of push-ups to feel that the effort was worth it. Sadie loves to get her stomach scratched and will get into position anytime I indicate I'll do this for her. While she is waiting for a stomach scratch, I'll do push-ups over her! Each time I lower myself to just above her, I am rewarded with a lick on the face. She never tires of this one either, ever hopeful that the stomach scratch will soon begin, which it does after I finish about ten push-ups.

Canine Calf Shapers

Sadie had previously interrupted all my efforts to do calf raises on the stairs. Now, I make her a part of the process, and it is great. I hold her under my arm for weight, and raise and perform the calf raise. Place your foot with the ball at the edge of the stair. Hold your dog under one arm, and hold on to the stair rail with the other. Raise and lower, feeling the stretch in your calf muscles. Repeat for each side.

Dog Leg Lifts

Sit on the couch or a chair with your feet flat on the floor in front of you. Allow your dog to straddle your legs and slowly lift your legs straight out in front of you. It's fun for your dog, and there's no danger of her getting hurt because you just raise her a few inches off the floor. You'll feel this working the backs of your thighs. It's a good replacement for the leg-curl machine, which I found extremely uncomfortable and unnerving, as I couldn't see who was laughing at me while my face was smashed into the bench of the machine.

Sock Slides

Have hardwood floors? This exercise gets both your floors and your legs in shape, and it's a game your dog will love. I have an old pair of thick socks I put on, and I slide sideways back and forth on the hardwood floors. This works the inner thigh muscle as you slide first one leg to the side and bring the other leg to meet it. Sadie loves chasing back and forth trying to keep up with me.

Dog Dancing

I'd never admitted it to anyone, but secretly, I love to dance. Forbidden to do so from a young age by some rigid religious reasoning from my parents, I'd never learned how. As I grew older, I envied the dancers I saw, but never got up the courage to take any lessons. Enter the partner I had been waiting for. In the confines of my house I started teaching myself how to dance with Sadie. With the oldies station blaring loudly, Sadie and I would dance in the dining room, through the living room and down the stairs to the basement.

We'd dance in the bedroom in the morning and a few quick steps in the kitchen after eating. It was fun, and she loved trying to keep up with me or jumped on me while I performed contortions I'd never have the nerve to do in front of anyone but Sadie. Dancing with your dog is fun: you burn calories, you laugh, you are energized.

All these exercises resemble the ones I attempted to do most of my adult life and was never able to keep up for very long. With Sadie, they were just part of the day. But Dogercise isn't limited to these specific routines—it's any activity that gets you moving and involves your dog. And trust me; the sky really is the limit on what you can do.

For example, just putting on my shoes some days involves a vigorous wrestling match. Sadie will grab one, and then I have to get it from her. In a simple wrestling session you are using your arm, leg, back and torso muscles.

You know that oversized beach ball that was supposed to transform your stomach into a pancake? Try using it with your dog. It's a lot of fun to take it into the backyard and roll around on it with your dog trying to jump on it. It hones your balance and works those abs and stomach muscles. You can teach your dog to jump over you while you're on the ball, which makes the exercise very interesting.

Take into account the endless times you have to get up and down to check on the dog when you'd normally be sitting doing nothing. Even when I'm trying to write, she finds ways to get me off the chair for periodic exercise. She'll come running with the rope chew and inevitably bang me in the ankle with it. If this has never happened to you, good, but for those of you it has happend to, you know that the pain is intense! A crack in the ankle from the knot in the rope toy necessitates getting up, applying ice to my ankle and, of course, taking a few minutes to throw it for her to bring to me, which inevitably leads to a game of tug-of-war. And did you know that if you walk around your house for just five minutes every hour during the day, you can burn an extra 200 to 300 calories a day? Now, you can either bank these into a calorie-burning account and lose some weight, or use it for justification for an ice-cream bar or some chocolate!

Dogercise is that quick sprint when you must escape the scene where your dog has unexpectedly taken a bathroom break. It's the struggle you have while holding her back from jumping on the mailman. It's the half hour you set aside to try some of the exercises I've described. Dogercise happens when you least expect it. A toy is placed on your lap, and you get up and play for ten minutes. Your dog disappears in the house and is strangely quiet so you go looking for her. It's that rush of adrenaline when she greets you after work, and the numerous times a week you must run the sweeper as she runs interference.

I finally found exercise that I can enjoy and not just endure. It doesn't cost me anything extra and requires nothing but a little time and Sadie. She never laughs at my efforts as I'm sure the members of my classes at the gym did, and I've met more men on my walks with Sadie than I ever met in the gym. I'm not an exercise physiologist, just someone who found activities that keep my body in reasonable shape while bringing a smile to my face.

I was thinner now, but I knew this was not why I was happier. I was living a new life, one I hadn't planned on, one that was given to me while I was unaware. Surely I had been out of my mind during those cold March nights I had to trek outside with this then-unnamed dog for her middle-of-the-night pee. Where had that unnamed dog gone, and when had she been replaced with this Sadie, my little canine soul mate who was an integral part of my life now? And what had happened to me? I was so much lighter in body and—it dawned on me—in spirit as well.

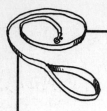

Dog Diet
DISCOVERIES

1. Whatever amount of time you have for physical activity is better than none at all.

2. Your dog will keep you active if you just follow her lead.

3. Exercise and endure are not synonymous!

4. Playing with your dog is a great way to keep in shape.

5. You and your dog can create your own fitness program. And, it can be fun.

PART TWO

Licking Stress
and Getting a
New Leash on Life

CHAPTER SEVEN

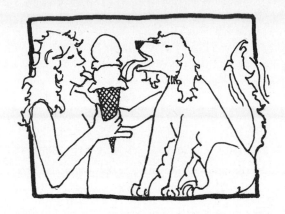

The Dog Ate My Diet

(Lame excuses for failure)

*A*s a former English teacher, I can tell you that anything you ever want to know about justifying failure, you learned in ninth grade. The excuses for lack of preparation in school easily carry over to every situation you'll encounter as you travel down the road of life. High school kids are masters at shrugging responsibility, and nothing is ever their fault. For example, I had to miss school one day and returned to find the notes left from my substitute describing my students as terrorists in training. Not only was I embarrassed and angry that they'd taken advantage of my absence and had made the substitute's day a living hell, but, if word got out, I was worried that I might not be able to get anyone to watch over this unruly bunch again.

For punishment, I assigned an essay asking my students to describe in great detail each and every thing that happened when I wasn't there. No one was allowed to stop writing until the bell rang. I'd teach them to behave like civilized human beings during my next departure from school. However, when reading their essays, I found only one student remotely admitted that anything had gone awry. He wrote, "Yes, we were bad, and we were rude, but other than that, we were good."

Over the years, that is the same reasoning I used to justify my trials and tribulations with diets. "Yes, I had two helpings of pasta, and I had tiramisu for dessert, but I didn't have whipped cream on the cappuccino." Or "Okay, I ate more of this container of ice cream than I'd planned, but I might as well finish it because it won't taste as good if I put it back in the freezer and it gets little ice crystals all over it." And how many of us have engaged in the faulty reasoning that we negated the calories from an overindulgent meal by sipping on a tasteless diet drink or a large glass of water with lemon? My all-time favorite is, "Well, I already blew it for today, but it wasn't my fault. How could I say no to that lunch invitation? How often do I get to eat there? I had to order their absolutely to-die-for mushroom pizza, and I could hardly turn down the free dessert. I'll just do better tomorrow." All those tomorrows just kept piling up along with the pounds. Until Sadie's arrival, that is. There are no excuses on the Dog Diet.

I was lucky. When Sadie ran into my house with her wisdom and voracious appetite, she helped me break bad habits and stop making excuses. Purportedly, it takes only three weeks to break a bad habit. Now, anyone who is firmly entrenched in self-destructive behavior knows that three weeks might as well be a lifetime. Almost all of the diets I had tried had a list of prohibited eating acts, and I was usually guilty of doing most of them. I'd tried reformation of various sorts, but only after Sadie brought these things to my attention did I actually see a way to eliminate my self-defeating rituals. One by one, I was able to identify the things that kept me back from what I wanted to achieve, and as they became apparent through my daily life with Sadie, I was able to change them, and you'll be able to do the same. Most likely you will recognize a little bit of yourself in some of these habits that follow. Ponder whether your excuses for perpetuating them aren't as silly as blaming lost homework on the dog.

Mindless Munching

In my experience almost all diet plans advocated taking the time to sit down and eat, taking your time to chew slowly and lots of other excellent tips. But I still used to love to eat in front of the television, read while eating or eat while surfing the Internet. My excuse for this was a sheer lack of time, and I could effectively accomplish two things at once. Unfortunately, while it saved time, it was totally ineffective toward my weight-control efforts.

Not only do you eat more if you eat while doing something else, you don't enjoy the food as much. It becomes a habit: noon news, sandwich; morning e-mail, bagel; suspenseful part of good book, ice cream. And then I'd go and have my "real" meal on top of this—the actual meal dictated by the specific diet I was cheating on at the time. I'd smugly eat the limited portions of tasteless food, completely ignoring the fact that I'd scarfed down untold calories while reading or watching television. When the scale didn't budge, I'd then have the excuse available that I'd eaten what the diet had recommended.

After Sadie's arrival, food had to be carefully guarded and eaten secretly, making eating while performing other activities nearly impossible. Not that I didn't try. While my food may have been within her reach when I ate in front of the television or reading in bed or on the sofa, she wasn't able to reach it while I ate at my desk. I realized I could hide a tempting dish behind my laptop screen, furtively reach around for a bite, and I was in hog heaven. That is, until the day a major mishap ended this decadent practice right along with the others.

I was done reading my e-mail and boldly finishing off a delicious bowl of clam chowder from one of my favorite restaurants. I clicked the "sign off" button and reached for the bowl at the same time the familiar "good-bye" chirped from the computer speaker. Sadie had come to realize that when she heard those words, I would be getting up, and it was her habit to stretch and come out from under the table.

Unfortunately, I hadn't noticed that she was lying beside my chair, and when she jumped up, she hit my arm, spilling remnants

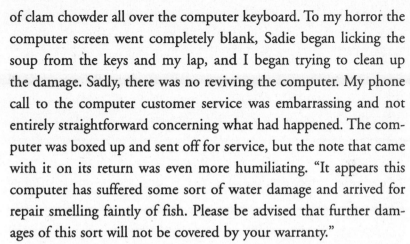

of clam chowder all over the computer keyboard. To my horror the computer screen went completely blank, Sadie began licking the soup from the keys and my lap, and I began trying to clean up the damage. Sadly, there was no reviving the computer. My phone call to the computer customer service was embarrassing and not entirely straightforward concerning what had happened. The computer was boxed up and sent off for service, but the note that came with it on its return was even more humiliating. "It appears this computer has suffered some sort of water damage and arrived for repair smelling faintly of fish. Please be advised that further damages of this sort will not be covered by your warranty."

Thus ended my eating in front of the computer as well as all the other activities I tried to include while eating unnecessary calories I thought didn't count, including a potato chip or two while on the treadmill. (Those small Pringles cans fit perfectly in the space intended for water bottles.) I thought they gave me that burst of energy needed to finish the workout. After all, wasn't I running off the calories just as soon as I swallowed them if I ate them on the treadmill? If I was going to quit these bad habits, I felt I might as well give them all up. And there were many—chocolate during a bubble bath, lunch while working and meals in the middle of the night when on business trips. (I just wanted to see if they were telling the truth when advertising twenty-four-hour room service.)

Sadie made it mandatory that eating was a solo activity in order to make sure that I was able to not only finish my meal, but that I didn't end up wearing it, destroying important electronic items or doubling my time spent exercising. I soon noticed that I had more

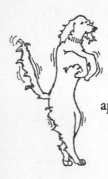

time for other activities, my dry cleaning bill was less and nothing had to be repaired or replaced due to something being spilled on it. Eating and only eating during mealtimes made a vast difference—my appetite and my waistline shrunk proportionately.

Cruising and Chewing

Another top diet buster for me was eating while in the car. I mistakenly believed that these calories didn't count either. I always felt like I was getting away with something as I ate on the sly, behind the wheel, on lonely stretches of interstate highways. In the early days with Sadie, I used my car as a sanctuary to wolf down fast food, but the truth is, I had always been defenseless against picking up fast food while traveling. It broke the monotony of an interstate trip and gave me the opportunity to try the many items I'd seen on late-night television commercials. If you think avoiding fast food would be easy with the dog in the car, it's just the opposite.

My own sense of smell is quite honed, but nothing compared to Sadie's. I first noticed her ability to ferret out fast-food joints before they were even in sight when we were on our way to Virginia Tech for a veterinary appointment with a cardiologist, Dr. Abbott. Sadie had been diagnosed with a troublesome heart condition, which necessitated that she see a specialist. Not that the condition bothered her one bit, though it certainly had me worried sick. She wasn't allowed to eat prior to the tests she was scheduled for; therefore, I felt I couldn't either. My empty stomach made its presence very clear as we approached an exit I knew was populated with eateries. I gritted my teeth knowing that I had to be strong and drive right past them. All the car windows were up, the sunroof closed, and still Sadie roused herself from her Dramamine-induced sleep to begin sniffing vigorously and licking the window. *How bad could it be,* I reasoned, *to quickly consume some hash browns and motor on down the highway?*

As I pondered this possibility, my car left the interstate seemingly on its own, and before I knew it I was at a drive-through window. Breakfast wasn't being served so I figured there wasn't much of a difference between hash browns and french fries, so what the heck. Wrong. For the first thing, hash browns, at least the McDonald's ones, are in one compact piece that can be eaten quickly, right from their paper holder. Not so with french fries. Ever the value-conscious consumer, I readily agreed to the offer for the supersize version.

As soon as the fries were in the car, all traces of the tranquilizing effect of Sadie's Dramamine were gone. She jolted to life, attacking the fries before I could even grab my change from the cashier. Fries went everywhere, even down the front of my shirt, as she tried to gobble them. I knew I'd have no explanation for the vet as to why I had allowed her to eat contrary to his specific instructions, so I tried to restrain her while maneuvering the car into a parking space where I could gather up the fries.

After parking, I snapped her leash on, got her out of the car and tethered her to a small tree. I shook the fries out from inside my shirt and gathered up all the fries from every nook and cranny in the front and backseat of the car. I was pleased to see that the super-size version really was a good value, but sadly I had to throw them all away. As I retrieved Sadie and wiped the traces of french fry grease off the seat, I noticed that at least four workers were crowded at the open window, and they were laughing along with the driver of the car that had been behind me. That was the last time I went through a fast-food restaurant pickup window while traveling—with or without Sadie; I had learned my lesson. Each time I was tempted, I remembered the french fry debacle, and just drove on by. I figure in a year's worth of driving, I've cut over a million calories out of my diet just by this simple change!

After-Work Weaknesses

Face it; after most of us finish our workday, we look for anything enjoyable. Whether it's a happy hour with free hors d'oeuvres or a feeding frenzy at our own refrigerator, we see food and refreshment at the end of the day, as reward or solace, or both. Sadie took care of both of these temptations for me and they were no longer an option on the Dog Diet.

Happy hours had been part of my daily schedule when I was a schoolteacher. There was a bar where most of my fellow faculty members congregated after school ended for the day. We'd water down our laments with two-for-one drinks and feed our fantasies of easier schedules, better-behaved students and bigger salaries with the free miniature pizzas, hot wings, fried cheese and other greasy munchies in the noisy bar. We'd demand silence from the students at lunchtime in the school cafeteria, then make almost as much noise as the out-of-control school cafeteria at these after-work gripe sessions.

About 6:00 P.M. I'd make my way home to go over lesson plans, check papers, watch television and eat my way through the rest of the evening. With that kind of calorie consumption, coupled with the school cafeteria food and the endless supply of doughnuts in the faculty room, my attempts to become slim had as much of a chance for becoming real as the fantasies we malcontent educators indulged in at happy hour.

Then I became a lawyer and attendance at happy hour was more of a requirement than a place to let off steam and wallow around with kindred spirits who endured the same daily mistreatment. These gatherings were an extension of the workday hours, filled with egotistical lawyers trying to outdo each other with war stories. While neither stress relieving nor a good time, these assemblies did somehow seem necessary, as they were times to network and keep abreast of what was going on and with whom. Besides, the free food at these dark-paneled lawyer bars was sumptuous, and the lack of lighting made it possible to place enough in my purse to have later at home.

Then Sadie arrived, and I was off the hook. She needed to go out immediately after work, not after a happy hour. I had a great excuse, and while I missed the food profoundly, I didn't miss the predatory crowd and was soon very glad to even be rid of the food, because it also erased the senseless calories I had sucked down day after day. Rushing home just to take Sadie out, put her back in her crate and run off to join the daily career comparisons at the watering hole wasn't an option. Sadie was much better company, and I am still grateful to her for curtailing my forays into the Tort Tavern where I was drowning in legal libations.

The after-work eating in front of the refrigerator ended as well. When I opened the front door each evening, the security alarm would chirp loudly, signaling my arrival home. This, in turn, triggered loud barking from Sadie in the basement, which caused me to scurry down the stairs and get her out immediately. For years, my habit had been to go straight to the refrigerator, get something to eat, retrieve my mail and eat while reading it.

With Sadie, I couldn't go to the refrigerator before getting her out of her crate as the barking was intolerable, and I couldn't go to it after I got her, because she'd want whatever I was trying to eat, plus she had to go out to the bathroom. In a short time, the after-work refrigerator dash was a practice of the past. I simply could not juggle all of Sadie's after-work activities *and* indulge in the refrigerator raid at the same time. Instead, if a cartoon like *Family Circus* depicted my footsteps through the house, it would go something like this: After coming through the front door, I go directly to the basement; I get Sadie out of her pennie and play a few games of toss with the pink chew bone, then we run up the steps; I don't hesitate in that dangerous area right outside the basement door where I could turn left and bolt to the refrigerator; I keep right on moving, avoiding the land mines of food within my easy grasp; I go upstairs and change my clothes quickly; return downstairs, actually bolting out the front door still avoiding the kitchen; and off we go on our walk. Thus, I steer clear of eating directly after work, and when we return, it's time for a Dog Diet dinner that we enjoy together!

Disastrous Dining

Pre-Sadie, each time I went out for dinner, I became the victim of some weird fatalistic thinking: *This might be the last time I eat at this particular restaurant. There could be a national ban on crème brûlée tomorrow. What if this could be my last meal . . . ever?* I've tried to figure out how this thinking developed, but for the life of me can't come up with anything definitive.

I was one of eight kids in a family where we never went to bed hungry, but with limited resources to tend to their large brood, my parents developed some frugal practices that I'm sure carried over to my adulthood in the form of always thinking that I needed to eat as much as possible when food was plentiful. These money-saving tactics included having us bend the truth about our age in order to get in on the free buffets at the rare restaurant we frequented. While traveling, my mom tried in vain to convince all of us that eating cold cereal and bologna sandwiches at roadside rest stops was an adventure, but it always made me just want to eat more and more when at last we'd get to eat dinner in a real restaurant.

Another possible reason is that as a single school-teacher living in the Washington, D.C., suburbs, I had little money left for food after paying rent and utilities, thus anytime I had a dinner date I

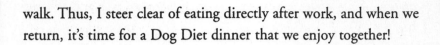

made sure I not only ate a lot, but had leftovers to take home. Of course, not having money for groceries did get me at the lowest weight of my life, except for the time I spent working in Guatemala where there was literally nothing to eat.

For whatever reason, when eating out, I was never able to order within reason or moderation, even if I was really trying to stick to a diet. When I was at a nice restaurant and someone else was picking up the check, I had no willpower whatsoever. It seemed like a stranger was spitting out my order for each and every thing on the menu that even had a hint of tasting great. Then Sadie put me through the wringer with food not only at home, but ruined my gluttonous escapades on someone else's tab. Instead of feeling free to order the most aromatic and noisy dish on the menu, I felt guilty because she was at home in her crate.

I simply couldn't enjoy whatever large repast was set before me. After eating a few bites, I was done. I'd take the rest home and eventually I'd share it with her. I discovered that eating out didn't have to mean overeating. I learned to order dishes consisting of the ingredients of meals I ate at home. These foods were healthy and lighter in calories. The dishes I began to enjoy were ones that I could share with Sadie and know that they were good for both of us. For example, now I'd order a large salad followed by grilled chicken, steamed brown rice and vegetables. It was a small sacrifice to order an entrée sans the fattening sauce described on the menu. To my delight, I found that eating out was a much more pleasant experience when I quit focusing solely on the food and more on my surroundings, noticing the ambiance of the restaurant, the table settings, the interesting people in the restaurant and the person across the table from me. And I didn't go home berating myself for eating too much or feeling bad for leaving Sadie at home. I started giving her the leftovers immediately when I returned home, thus avoiding the temptation of a trip to the refrigerator in the middle of the night. It worked. I kept getting slimmer, I didn't feel guilty and, unlike in the past, first dinner dates with men weren't the last. They could actually afford to take me out more than once.

Flyby Feasting

Flyby feasting reminds me of the brief appearances stunt pilots make at air shows. The acrobatic planes appear out of nowhere, perform a few maneuvers, then they're gone as the exhaust smoke lingers in the sky. Flyby feasting, also known as eating on the run, is similar. You just buzz by the samples attractively displayed in the supermarket, taking a bite of this and a bite of that or grabbing a handful of nuts while waiting for a take-out order at the bar, but the exhaust fumes from your whirlwind performance present themselves as extra calories, and unlike the residue from the stunt planes, which eventually dissipates, these remain as extra pounds.

Eating on the run is different from eating while driving. I'm talking about the days when you have a hectic schedule and don't sit down to take the time to eat—when you grab this and that, grazing your way until evening, when to your surprise you're ravenous. You've consumed hollow calories all day that have none the less added up to more than a day's allotment, but still you eat more.

Eating on the run is all the mindless calories you consume while shopping. A chocolate chip cookie here, an ice-cream cone there, samples of every fattening processed food your supermarket offers. It's the junk that you just *have to have* at a street fair or a carnival. Eating on the run is grabbing that doughnut on the receptionist's desk as you enter your office, or anything else that someone has placed there because they don't want it. Dogs can't eat on the run. They have to stand at their dish and finish their meal. Sadie taught me to slow down, eat when I was supposed to and let it be.

Before Sadie, breakfast was a hit-or-miss event depending on how much time I had in the morning. Despite the fact that I knew it was the most important meal of the day, I held on to the belief that if I missed eating in the morning, it wasn't a big deal. I also thought it perfectly fine to eat whatever was left in the refrigerator from the night before, *plus* any prescribed item for the particular diet plan I was trying at the time.

It was always on days that started out with a missed breakfast that things went downhill. I'd get hungry midmorning and need a muffin from the vending machine or some of the candy I had hidden in my desk. These were the days I grabbed lunch on the go while on the way to a meeting, or I had to eat at my desk.

Eating at my desk always resulted in eating more than I planned because in order to get something delivered, we all know you have to order a certain amount. This minimum order requirement always resulted in a maximum amount of food that I would polish off during the course of the afternoon. Dinner would be a continuation of the same, and I'd end my day feeling bloated and defeated.

Sadie required a lot of tending during those early blurry days of feedings, walks, fighting over food, bathroom breaks and barking. However, what happened when I wasn't paying attention (because I was usually too tired or too hungry to notice) was that we developed a schedule. Breakfast was at a certain time, followed by lunch and dinner. Not that you could set your watch by us, but our mealtimes became regular and my life more organized. I was able to have a decent idea of what I'd eaten at the end of the day because I hadn't grabbed things here and there throughout the day.

I started taking Sadie with me to street fairs and festivals where food was in abundance. With her along, I wasn't able to go to the food booths, because they didn't allow dogs. I was able to enjoy all the sights and events without gaining an ounce thanks to her. She'd sniff happily as we wound through craft tables, listened to music, sorted through old books for sale and enjoyed other activities that before had always been accompanied by food. I became mindful of all my eating, and in doing so, quit eating on the run, which enabled me to lighten up on having to run all those calories off later.

Office Parties and Food Bullies

Everyone tries to avoid the office drunk at office parties. Their obnoxious behavior is almost unbearable, plus if they glom on to you, who knows what the rumors will be around the workplace after the party. However, for the diet-conscious, there is a worse party animal out there, and that's the "food bully."

Food bullies try to make you eat everything and anything. "Try it," they coax. If that doesn't work, they try to flatter you into eating by saying, "You don't have to watch your figure, go on have some." I've even had these bullies actually put food on my plate and refill my glass despite my protests. I'll take the office drunk over the food bully any day.

As Sadie and I developed the eating plan for the Dog Diet, I realized that I was a combination of both of these characters when it came to how I treated food. I not only overindulged like the office drunk, I was a food bully—to myself. I used many of these same arguments to justify my own indulgences; I was as bad as the woman at a party who actually tried to feed me a large bite of her peach cobbler. And there wasn't much difference between me and the guy who had to be cut off from the open bar at a Christmas party. When it came to food, I just didn't know my own limits.

Through the development of my eating plan with Sadie, I saw that food wasn't the most important part of the day or my life anymore. The results of regulated eating, of planning ahead, freed me from indulging. I'd watch Sadie give up and go eat her own food when she'd discover what I was eating wasn't something she was interested in, and it encouraged me to do the same with foods that weren't good for me.

Now when I am confronted with a food bully, I'm sweetly resolute in refusing. I picture Sadie when I try to give her medications or vitamins. It's a struggle, and I don't always succeed in getting her to swallow them. I picture this person holding me by the hair and forcing my mouth open as they pop the food morsel in and then massage my throat to get me to swallow it. That's just not going to happen, but the vision has saved me many needless and unnecessary calories at social events. If my firm, but polite, resolve doesn't work, I tell them I've just gotten over a twenty-four-hour virus and have eaten some of everything at the party, but feel certain that I'll start vomiting again if even one more crumb of food goes into my mouth! Trust me, this causes the toughest of food bullies to slink away, taking the unwanted food with them.

Licking Your Plate Clean

Almost everyone I know was told while growing up that they had to eat everything on their plate. We've all been regaled with tales of starving children in Africa and how ungrateful we are if we waste food. Is it any wonder that most of us are overweight, haunted by these childhood warnings that cause us yet today to eat everything put in front of us? Over the years, I thought this was a most excellent excuse for my overeating. After all, my inner child was telling me it didn't want to leave anything behind as my outer self got bigger and bigger, and it just wasn't my fault.

I don't think dogs are told this same tale by their mothers. If anything, their mothers are most likely exhausted from the entire litter helping themselves to breakfast, lunch and dinner, and are relieved if the puppies eat as little and as quickly as possible. That must have been the case in Sadie's family. Except for the first night Sadie came to my home, she never ate everything in her dish. I know one of her reasons for this had to be that she was holding out for some of my food, but I also know that she just liked to go back later and finish it off. This is a great method for controlling your own calorie intake.

I choose a reasonable amount of the food that will not make me feel stuffed from the Dog Diet food list, arrange them artfully on my plate, then I try not to eat everything. I like saving a little of it for later on, knowing I'm not eating any more calories than I'd intended to eat to begin with. Then if I want a snack, I can have it without feeling guilty.

If you're having a salad meal, don't put the dressing on all of it at once. Just put dressing on half the salad and save the other half if you are no longer hungry. That way it doesn't get all soggy, and you can even have the variety of choosing a different dressing. If all you have left over is rice and vegetables, these can be reheated together, and some dried cranberries added to them can almost fool you into thinking it's a dessert.

Saving part of your dinner or lunch can become a challenge to use it as a snack later in a creative manner. Remember, these snacks are all foods that your dog won't detect, and you can enjoy them a second time in peace. Leftover chicken or other meat can be wrapped in a tortilla with mustard and lettuce for a quick pick-me-up midafternoon. Cottage cheese can be mixed with applesauce for a sweet treat. Even an omelet from breakfast can be reheated and topped with salsa midmorning to get over a slump. Let your imagination be your guide. Remember that we were told many myths in childhood that most likely weren't true, including the one about cleaning your plate. Think about it; did you ever really see the Tooth Fairy or the Easter Bunny?

Dieting Delayed

In James Bond's world, tomorrow may never die, but in the world of dieting, tomorrow never comes. Believe me; I've started more diets tomorrow than anyone. Two phrases that will kill your attempts to get in shape are:

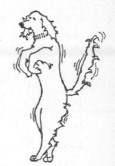

1. I'll do it later.
2. I'll start tomorrow.

There are consequences to delay, and I realized this full force as I learned to care for Sadie. Dogs can't wait to be taken care of. They can't just go get their own water or take themselves for a walk. They can't open their food or mix it in the bowl. They depend on us to be there when they need something. I can't tell Sadie that I'll take her outside tomorrow or that I'll feed her next week. Similarly, we need to be there for ourselves.

If you decide to wait until tomorrow to eat better and healthier, there will just be new temptations to deal with. It seems every day something new is invented that sounds so good. You could go on and on tasting new things, waiting until tomorrow, and never get yourself on a healthier eating plan.

While people are quick to shove food at us, or take us to nice restaurants with delicious food, only we are responsible for what actually goes into our mouths, and when we decide to take responsibility for it. There really is no time like the present. I had years of on-and-off again dieting until this little dog made me realize the importance of right now.

It's the same for getting more active. How many times did you tell yourself in the morning that you'd exercise or go for a walk later that day? How many times did you fail to do it? If you're like me, probably more times than you care to remember. With Sadie, I have no choice but to get up and out in the morning. I have to walk her at noon and again in the evening. Even with those walks as a minimum, I'm doing more than I did when I continually put things off. Weight—it just can't wait! Get on with it!

Snacks Before Sleeping

I loved to eat before bed. For a long time in my life, a turkey sandwich on rye was almost an aphrodisiac to me. This came to a screeching halt when Sadie became my roommate.

When I was a kid, my dad loved to give us cereal, ice cream or homemade milkshakes before we went to bed. I have warm memories of sitting at the picnic table in our kitchen with my brothers and sisters watching Dad prepare these treats. It was a ritual I carried with me when I went to college and beyond.

College dorms are notorious for late-night eating, and I was right in the thick of it—always in on any pizza order or late-night popcorn feasts. After graduation, I carried on the tradition in my first apartment, and when I got married, my husband and I would often have a glass of wine and a snack before retiring.

One of the diet plans I tried to follow advocated a snack before bed, and I was thrilled until I discovered the snack could be either cottage cheese or scrambled egg whites, not turkey sandwiches or milkshakes. I slugged through scrambled egg whites before retiring, believing the theory that if I didn't, my body would think it was starving during the night and hold on to all the extra calories I'd consumed during the day instead of burning them up. Even so, my body must not have gotten the message, because I still woke up hungry in the morning.

With Sadie, I developed a comfortable truce to the late-night snacks. Instead of depriving myself, I substituted my snack with a selection from the Dog Diet while Sadie ate the few bites saved from her dinner still left in her food bowl. I'd have an orange and a small piece of cheese—okay, I *had* to share the cheese with Sadie. An apple and a small amount of cottage cheese was also a satisfying snack and caused no increase in my weight. Sometimes Sadie has a Frosty Paws and I have a low-calorie fudge bar while we sit together on the steps, and yes, sometimes I do pretend it's a turkey sandwich.

Love Like Chocolate

Yep, the biggest excuse I ever had for eating too much, being lazy and lying around was the one we all know about: feeling sad, bad, nervous or happy. You name the emotion, I've eaten to get through it. And if I couldn't have mashed potatoes, there was always chocolate to provide a temporary Band-Aid for my wounded heart or to help me celebrate.

Sadie showed me what comfort really means. She's happy in the morning. She's happy in the evening. Although she sometimes sulks when I have to leave her, her joy at my return is constant. I've furtively peaked through the basement window at her in her crate when she didn't know I was there. I didn't see a frantic dog chewing on everything in sight. I saw a peaceful dog occupying herself with a toy or watching her television.

I've rested in the comfort and consistency of Sadie's devotion to me, and it has helped me to overcome emotional eating. She made it possible for me to quit hungering over love in the form of approval from others. Sure, she almost starved me to death in the beginning, but hey, look where it got me!

Happiness isn't a condition; it's a decision. I've learned from my wonderful dog that each day we should just decide to be happy, and we will be. She doesn't wait to see what I say or do to her in the morning before she starts thumping her tail on the bed. She's just happy.

If I'm in a hurry and don't have time to give her as much attention as I should, she doesn't run to her food dish and eat everything in a hurry. If she can't find her lobster or her tennis ball, she doesn't sit longingly in front of the drawer where her treats are. The winter of my discontent, when I tried to eat and drink my way through the grief of a lost romance, I only succeeded in making myself feel worse. I wasn't eating when my body was hungry, but when my heart was. That's not only why I gained weight that winter, but why I had been unable to ever successfully keep weight off for any length of time. Over the years I kept taking more and more of what I could get, which was food, because I could never get enough of what I wanted in the form of love, or joy, or self-worth or contentment. Who knew a little dog with all her antics and needs could show me that filling myself up with empty calories would only fill me out!

Why are foods we find solace in always so fattening? For myself, I blame my mother, because my first memory of food as comfort comes from her. When I was sick as a child, she would mash potatoes and carrots together, slather them with butter and serve me as much as I wanted. It was a supernatural elixir that always made me feel better. Even on television and in movies, foods people use for consoling themselves are the most calorie-laden. Remember *Beverly Hills 90210?* Those characters rushed to the Peach Pit for a generous helping of peach pie to ease the pain of their tumultuous love lives. Of course, on the show they all remained rail thin thanks to the illusion of television. What about the movies where the characters drown their sorrows in booze or eat all their meals at four-star restaurants, never exhibiting one ounce of added weight?

For once I'd like to see someone rush to the refrigerator upon receiving bad news and stuff their face with a tossed salad. Why can't a bag of carrots impart the same soothing effect as a box of chocolate? Why do policemen always belly up to the counter for doughnuts when beset by a perplexing crime? Why don't they just have a serving of cottage cheese? I can't think of one low-calorie, healthy food I ever resorted to, to ease pain or help me celebrate.

Emotions are fleeting, but the effects from the food we stuff ourselves with to overcome them can be permanent. Broken hearts, no matter how shattered, eventually become whole again. Anger fades

away, today's celebration is soon forgotten, but when we stuff ourselves with pizza and chocolate over them, we aren't allowing ourselves to really feel what we were intended to experience. We cover
things up, and soon we are covered in a layer of fat that we try forever to get rid of while eating more and more to feel less and less.

Here's what I often say to Sadie when she's about to wrestle free
from me during her bath or jump on a visitor, "Don't do it, Sadie,"
and I've come to say it to myself when I'm tempted to block out
some feeling I don't want to feel by eating. "Don't do it, Pat," I say,
and then I laugh because Sadie looks at me like I'm crazy for talking to myself. I let the mood take its course, and I have truly
learned that nothing can be assuaged forever by a trip to the refrigerator. Remember the saying, "Don't wear your heart on your
sleeve"? How about not wearing your failures, your successes, your
broken hearts, your anger, your disappointments, your jubilation
. . . on your hips?

These aren't all the excuses for failing at dieting, but they're a
good start for you to recognize your own reasons for starting over
again and again and never getting anywhere. In various unintentional ways, Sadie taught me all about excuses. If you pay attention,
your dog will do the same for you.

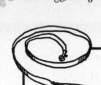

Dog Diet

DISCOVERIES

1. Anything worth doing is worth doing right now.

2. Excuses are easy, and ridiculous ones are endless.

3. Chocolate melts, so if you use it to mend your heart, it won't last.

4. Anything worth eating is worth eating well.

5. Conscious eating beats mindless munching in every way.

6. Eating doesn't fill you up . . . it fills you out!

CHAPTER EIGHT

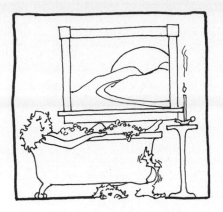

Living in the Moment

(Don't tug on your leash)

Dogs aren't the only creatures controlled by leashes. Sure, dogs' leashes are tangible and visible, but the ones that control human beings are less real. While one of the first obedience school lessons dogs learn is not to tug on their leashes, most people never master this. Sadie was no different than most dogs; she tugged and pulled on her leash when first learning to walk with me. This had an immediate consequence: she choked herself. The more she tugged on the leash, the tighter her collar became and the harder it was for her to breathe without choking and gagging.

It didn't take long for her to realize that if she allowed a little slack on the leash, she wouldn't hurt herself and could breathe freely while enjoying her walk. Why can't we learn to "give ourselves some slack"?

Unlike dogs', humans' leashes are invisible, and the negative results of tugging on them aren't immediately manifested. The restrictions we push ourselves to overcome nonetheless eventually have consequences. The one common restraint we all have on our lives is that of time. As the old saying goes, "Time and tide wait for no man." No matter how rich or poor, how heavy or thin, no one has more hours or minutes in the day than anyone else. Yet we tug and pull at these minutes and hours, wanting them to go faster or to be longer so we can cram more and more into them.

Today it's considered quite an enviable accomplishment to be a multitasker. If you can take care of business deals on your cell phone while driving your car, listening to the radio and eating lunch, you're doing fine. If you've got dinner preparations going, laundry in the washer, news on the television and can check your e-mail and apply nail polish all at the same time, more power to you. The sad fact about this multitasking world is that we've purposely chosen to speed up our lives and crowd so much into one day that doing more than one thing at a time becomes a necessity.

During my early weeks with Sadie, I felt like I was just flying through all the tasks of my life in order to get them all done, plus care for her, all in the same amount of time I'd had just to take care of myself before she came to live with me. I seemed to have no downtime, but then when I looked at her, she was never frazzled, never rushed, never doing two things at once. Never did I see her eating and playing with her rope toy at the same time. Not once did she bring along an unfinished rawhide chew on her walk or lick my face while surreptitiously watching Animal Planet. She seemed to be able to get through her days doing one thing at a time, but I'd never done that.

No, if I was reading, I was most likely eating. If I was watching television, I was most often reading and eating. Even caring for Sadie, sometimes I'd talk on my cell phone while walking her and try to sneak in a bite or two of a missed meal, or read the newspaper in between tosses of the tennis ball. And I'd always been one to speed through things I didn't really want to do, like cleaning the house or sessions on the treadmill.

We have all wished that certain moments would hurry by, but in doing this, we've also rushed through hours and days. Some of the longest moments and hours of my life were those early days of Sadie's incessant barking and begging for food. Each night seemed endless as I hoped and prayed it would go quickly and I'd get some sleep. Every meal was approached with optimism that I'd be able to eat quickly before she noticed. I spent way too much time wishing these moments away, and then, they were over.

Looking back, it seemed like those times were only a blur. Somewhere in those moments that I was wishing away, the barking stopped, mealtimes were no longer a struggle, and the little curly-eared puppy had turned into a skinny, long-legged Pollyanna who followed me everywhere. I couldn't imagine living without her, and I was sorry that I'd let so many of the moments slip by—I'd tugged on my leash, and I regretted it.

I promised myself that I would no longer live out of the moment. I'd taken Sadie's astute advice, and I'd gotten lighter, learned how to let go of past hurts, how to eat better, how to keep my mental and physical metabolism going at a steady pace, and now it was time to learn to slow down. I'd learned that getting rid of a heavy body involved much more than what I did or didn't put in my mouth. I was seeing that when I began to lighten up my thinking, my body had gotten lighter. I marveled at the paradox that my life had become much more active with Sadie; I'd revved my body into a superefficient exercise machine, while the pace of my life had simultaneously slowed down—all these factors together had helped me get thinner. I realized, however, that more important than the spectacular weight loss, one of the greatest lessons Sadie taught me was to live in, not out of, the moment.

We live out of the moment when we think ahead, spend time regretting the past or don't take the time to pay attention to what is going on in our lives *right now*. Living out of the moment is hurrying past a beautiful sunset, rushing through the morning and fretting the time away when we're stuck in traffic.

For chronic dieters, which of course includes me, living out of the moment is the eternal hope we have that tomorrow will be different, coupled with an intense belief that someday we will again look like we once did. It's paying no attention to the moment we eat that serving of mashed potatoes, forgetting that we already had the "one" piece of chocolate we allotted ourselves for today. It's a cultivated lack of conscious responsibility for our food world in general. In dieting, as in life, we have lots of leashes holding us back from certain food items and activities, but we constantly tug on them "just this once." Tugging on my good eating leash "just this once" put extra pounds on me time and time again. Once I learned not to tug on my leash, much the same way as Sadie had, I no longer needed to rush through my day, I was able to give complete concentration to what I was doing at the moment, and it made my days longer and my waistline smaller.

If you think this won't help you, doesn't apply to weight loss and that you aren't guilty of living out of the moment, take this simple test. Get a blank sheet of paper. Try to answer these questions:

1. What was the first thing I thought about when I woke up today?
2. What did I see when I looked out the window this morning?
3. Who was the first person I talked to today and what about?
4. How many times did I say "thank you" today?
5. What made me smile today?
6. Did I hear any music today that brought back a memory?
7. What specific tastes do I remember from today?
8. What did I think about today? Was there a moment my mind was empty?
9. How did I decide what to wear this morning?
10. What will I remember about today?

If you can't remember the individual moments, tastes, sounds, people and events that made up your day, you need to slow down and take a look at what you do with your time.

These are the things that make up the moments of your day, and your days make up the weeks of your life. Then the weeks make up the months and then the years, and it all becomes a blur, except for the special moments you chose to live to the fullest, to savor and to make a memory of. But if you are constantly tugging on your leash, you won't emerge from the missed moments as Sadie did, a skinny, long-legged dog that enjoys each bite of her food, each round of play with her toys and every walk. You'll be like I was, a round, discontented person, regretful that the moments slipped away. Your moments will have meant nothing to you, and your dissatisfaction with yourself will be everything.

Sadie took pleasure in each activity that she was involved in. When she ate, she did so heartily, licking her lips and wriggling in delight at some particularly flavorful bite. When she napped, she was out cold, and when she was held or petted, she reveled in the attention. I started experiencing the activities of my own life with more intensity and appreciation. All of our lives are different, but we share many similar "moments" during the day. When you take the time to savor them, routine activities can become special events. As I watched Sadie, and our lives became intertwined as we developed the Dog Diet, most days I quit tugging on my leash. I saw how to lighten up my life by living in the moment, and you can too.

The Morning Moment

Why do we all rush through the morning? If there's a comic strip character I could relate to, it was Dagwood (from *Blondie*) and his eternal scramble to get to work on time. Most mornings were a blur—a part of my day that had to be endured, most often faced as late as possible and gotten through as quickly as possible. When Sadie was still sleeping in her crate in the basement, she wanted mornings to come as quickly as possible so she could get out of there. Her barks began before the sun was shining and caused me to hide under the covers.

However eager she was for her morning to begin, she was in no hurry to rush it along. Nope, she took her time with everything and clearly enjoyed each and every event of her morning. While she would dash out the front door and both of us would run to the boulevard where we walked, once there, she was in no hurry. Sadie took the time to notice ducks on the river, the man painting his mailbox, the bottle of beer left on the riverbank by a drunk the night before, and, of course, she sniffed out any carelessly discarded fast-food wrappers. She'd face the bright morning sun, squinting her eyes, nipping an interesting blade of grass and carefully observing a squirrel. She'd often become so filled with utter joy that to express this, she'd stop to stand on her hind legs and playfully hit me with her paws.

I soon was treasuring my morning moments as well. Don't wait to see how the day turns out; predestine all your days to be happy ones by having a great attitude about the day ahead. Take a moment to relax, sip your coffee and savor its taste. Eat a nice breakfast and read the paper. If you think you don't have time, get up earlier or chop some fruit the night before and arrange it nicely on a plate. It's a welcome and cheerful sight when you open the refrigerator the next morning.

Take time to get ready for work. If it's a dark and dreary day, pick a bright-colored article of clothing. If it's cold, wear some tropical-smelling perfume. If it's warm and the sun is shining, be grateful. When you leave your house for work, your morning won't be a blur of hurried activities, but a pleasant feeling that you lived in the moment. You'll have a feeling of self-satisfaction; that everything is right in your world. I imagine my day as a blank page of paper, and I want the first entries to be clear activities that set the tone for my day, not a bunch of hasty ink smudges I can barely read.

Remember the mornings of the calorie-laden breakfasts? Eggs Benedict used to be my favorite. This breakfast, along with other indulgent ones like hotcakes and syrup or cheese- and bacon-laden omelets, always made my day get off to a sluggish start. None of these breakfasts are possible on the Dog Diet, so a heavy breakfast is no longer a problem. However, heavy thoughts in the morning, frantic rushing to get everything done—these will weigh down your day and set in motion a day that is not the best it could have been.

Now I start my mornings laughing while I have a tongue-lick facial applied before my feet ever hit the floor, followed by a healthy, light breakfast, and I am off and running, but not at the speed of sound. Morning moments are the first steps to a memorable day. Be happy for another day of life, and look forward to the challenges the day might bring. Prepare for them with the foundation you build with your morning moments.

Magic Moments

Magic moments are moments that can never be duplicated. Miss them and they are gone forever. Like soap bubbles that evaporate before your eyes, they're a one-shot deal. Magic moments will happen if you take the time to allow them to happen.

I learned about magic moments from Sadie. She'd be lying on the floor and notice something outside the front door. Quickly, she'd go to the door and just watch whatever had caught her attention. If we were eating in the backyard and a fly landed on her food, she'd lower her head and follow its every motion until her nose got too close and it flew away. She was fascinated with anything unexpected that came into her view and took the time to observe it.

Years ago, I had rented a small apartment in a large house owned by a couple in their late eighties. When the husband was giving me the tour of the property, he told me there was one rule that he expected all his tenants to follow: we must stop and smell the roses—and he meant it. He cultivated beautiful roses of every variety and hue and wanted to share their beauty with us.

After I bought my house, I planted a number of roses in the backyard, but in the initial years as a property owner I gave them little notice, until Sadie brought them to my attention. She loved them, and even when she was just a little puppy, she would stand on her hind legs to sniff them. I'd sit at the table in my backyard and watch her as she went from one rosebush to the next, her delicate little nose sniffing the subtle differences in the fragrances. This was a magic moment.

A magic moment is the small patch of color in a vast asphalt parking lot where one wildflower has dared to poke up through a crack in the pavement. It's that feeling of accomplishment when you complete an overwhelming project. It's the afternoon sun shining on the water (even if it's just a mud puddle). It's the sweet face of a little child pressed up against the window in the car next to you in traffic. It's that moment when you get into bed at night, and your entire body just relaxes, and you feel safe and warm.

Sadie and I time many of our walks to coincide with when the sun will set on the river we walk by. It's always beautiful, and rather than lament that another day of my life has passed and maybe I don't have the perfect life, I treasure this moment. Standing there with my little dog, I recall the other magic moments I've taken the time to appreciate during the day. I stare into the rays of sunlight reflecting off the river and pretend they are washing over me like a refreshing shower that energizes me for the evening ahead. I feel satisfied walking home, and it has nothing to do with what I've eaten that day.

Of course, I have days that spill over with runs in my panty hose, food spilled on blouses, phone calls I need to return and even a bill or two that's overdue. I lose the car keys, forget to use waterproof mascara and work with people who get on my nerves. That's life. But taking pleasure in the magic moments enables you to glide over all the other things that are annoying or disturbing. Magic moments make us feel lighter and validate that we *are* lighter. Don't miss them because you're too busy doing something else. A lighter mind from a day of noticing magic moments makes a lighter body—give it a try.

"Me" Moments

"Me" moments are the times during the day you reserve just for yourself. These are essential for a lighter mind and should comprise only light thoughts, light food or light activities. "Me" moments don't have to be planned and can be enjoyed anywhere.

Contrary to what you may have heard from family or friends who are good at making us feel guilty about the time we need to ourselves, time alone is not selfish time. I grew up in a noisy home with seven siblings. Add to the din of all these kids a mother who believed with all her heart that "idle hands were the devil's workshop," and anyone would've run screaming from the house for a moment of inactivity and silence. I developed quite a scheme back then to escape this palace of productivity fate had sentenced me to.

I created hand-loomed pot holders and sold them over the countryside from the back of my horse. My mom was satisfied with my industrious endeavors, and since she didn't want to purchase all of them, it was a feasible excuse for me to slip away on sales trips with my horse, Misty. With a favorite book, a blanket, an egg salad sandwich and no intentions of spending the whole day peddling pot holders, I'd ride off on my horse to a favorite secluded field. Once there, Misty would drift away to munch on summer clover, and I'd lie under the bright summer sun feeling like I was in heaven. I'd read and dream and often fall asleep. I'd return to the house rested, having escaped to a different world.

So, long before Sadie came into my life, I knew these moments were important. As an adult, I'd even been to a spa in Arizona that specializes in teaching busy women the importance of taking time out for themselves and living in the now. As I rode in the desert on horseback, I remembered the many times I'd ridden away on Misty, vowing that when I returned home I'd spend more time doing activities just for me. Once I was back in my hectic world, I'd soon forget the lessons learned at Miraval.

Sadie became a daily reminder for taking "me" moments—she did it all the time! She was an expert at taking the shortest of naps, but sleeping deeply. She'd take time to just sit looking out the front door and would groom her paws for the longest time. I've gotten very few manicures because I've always felt I just couldn't take the time to do it unless I could drop my hands off at the salon while I went to the office.

During the development of the Dog Diet, there were days I was totally exhausted and the fatigue alone forced me to take "me" moments. Over time, I've found that there really is time for me, and I make sure to take it.

I've created a comfort corner in my home where I spend many of these moments. It's a little room right off the kitchen, which prior to the Dog Diet would have been dangerous territory, but now is just perfect. I'm even in plain sight of the refrigerator but able to concentrate on what my moment is all about instead of what's to eat!

This room was just sitting there waiting for a useful purpose when I decided to create a little place in my house just for me to enjoy. I found a darling little wicker sofa with a matching coffee table on sale, and they fit perfectly in the room. I painted the walls a bright, tropical color and displayed my many souvenirs from my vacations at the beach. I filled a corner china cabinet with special dishes and cups to use for tea. I added a small tropical-motif throw rug, and there I had it—a cozy retreat.

It is here, surrounded by lovely items that bring back wonderful memories, that I take the time to have moments for myself every day. Sometimes my moments are infused with sunlight from the window that looks out on my yard, and other times they're spent by candlelight. Even if you don't have a spare room to make into your own personal-moment sanctuary, you can make a special area in another room just for you. It can be a comfortable chair next to a window or fireplace. Just find any little space that you can carve out just for yourself, and it won't cost a lot of money to buy a few special items to place there as well as other treasures you already have.

"Me" moments aren't always just sitting in a special place and taking the time to do something for myself; they can be other things that you find pleasure in.

1. Enjoy a nice cup of tea. (I bought a very thin bone china cup at a flea market. I use this cup in my special room, and yes, I do think the tea tastes better from it.)
2. Soak your feet in warm water with some aromatic bath salts.
3. Listen to relaxing music.

4. Read those magazines you subscribe to but never open.

5. Take the time to write a handwritten note of appreciation to someone.

6. Take a nap.

7. Be a tourist in your own town. Take a few hours to visit a tourist attraction, and have lunch just as if you were from somewhere else.

8. Buy yourself some flowers.

9. Plan a week's worth of menus.

10. Watch a movie without doing anything else.

11. Buy a really nice set of sheets with the highest thread count you can afford. You'd be surprised at the great quality sheets now available at discount stores.

12. Put photos from your last vacation in a nice album.

13. Make a Christmas or birthday wish list of things *you* would like to have.

14. Experiment with different candle and incense fragrances. See what gives you energy, calms you down and so on.

15. Do nothing. That's right—*nothing*. Just sit and let your mind and body totally relax.

How do these activities fit in with the Dog Diet? You are no longer focused on what you're going to eat or seeking comfort by filling your stomach. These activities are part of the new lighter mind-set you are cultivating to go along with your lighter body.

The Mundane Moments

Taking a dog outside to the bathroom was not something I'd ever thought would be a part of my daily routine. Each day we all have a myriad of things to do that certainly aren't exciting, but they *must* be done anyway. I call these the mundane moments.

When you allow your thoughts to be lighter, you develop the ability to not get bogged down in the daily details. Sadie was fascinated by everything I did. From the sound of the hair dryer, to the noises from the coffee machine, to the preparation of the most meager form of sustenance . . . everything was interesting to her. Not everything in life can be fun, let alone exciting, but Sadie's fascination with my routines made me take a new look at some of them, and in doing so I made them more enjoyable. Now, I haven't found an entertaining way to clean the toilet bowl or to laugh myself silly sweeping up dog hair, but some mundane things can be done in a lighter manner. Here are a few things almost all of us have to take time to do. Some are just time-consuming; some we allow to cause stress, which makes us want to eat!

1. Brushing teeth: Use a new flavored toothpaste. From vanilla mint to cinnamon these new flavors take away the monotony and make you not want to eat soon afterward.

2. Washing sheets: I discovered wonderful linen rinses at one of my favorite discount stores. Lavender is great to rinse your sheets in, but my favorite is a mint-rosemary scent. I'm still searching for one that makes them smell like they were dried outside.

3. Makeup: I put the change from my pockets and the bottom of my purse in a pretty dish on my dresser each night. At the end of the month, I have enough change to buy a Chanel lipstick. It's less fattening than chocolate and always adds a spark to my day.

4. Ironing: I just don't do it. Seriously, I have always hated to iron, and now I don't do it at all. Permanent press was made for me, and wrinkled clothes are a fashion statement.

5. Dog bath: I just grit my teeth, put on some old clothes, add some lively music and make it into a Dogercise session.

6. Bedtime: Start your rituals a little earlier so you're not so tired. Have a low-calorie snack with your dog, slip into those freshly laundered and fragrant sheets and allow yourself to just settle into a relaxing night's rest.

7. Work: Take a moment each day to think about what you do. Make a notation on your calendar of one thing you're proud of accomplishing. Give a compliment (at least a semi-sincere one) to a disagreeable coworker.

8. Filling the car up with gas: I hate smelling like gasoline, and I always succumb to the temptations of the worst supposedly edible items on the counter when I go in to pay. Now I keep a pair of garden gloves in my trunk to wear when pumping gas, and I pay at the pump, so I avoid the food traps inside the station.

9. Waiting in lines: Try to never buy more that twenty items at one time, and you can always go through the express. At banks, use the drive-through, and for anything else, try to

find a store that's open twenty-four hours so you can go in the middle of the night.

10. Taking out the trash: I've tricked Sadie into thinking that dragging the bag to the curb is a game.

Mealtime Moments

A lighter body and lighter way of thinking brings on a lighter way of eating, but it doesn't mean you don't get to enjoy mealtimes anymore. The kitchen is often the social center of the house, and many special mealtime moments can be part of the Dog Diet. Once you have your kitchen stocked with the food on the list and your Salad Box in place, mealtime moments will be wonderful, not a confusion of "what can I eat?" You will find delight in preparing all your meals and use this time as a chance to talk and laugh with friends, family and your dog.

When we gather to celebrate or mourn, food is front and center. When I was growing up, we ate dinner together every night. Attendance at the evening meal was mandatory, and everyone was grilled about their school day, how much homework they had (you had to answer this cautiously as your answer governed the remainder of your evening) or if they'd finished their chores. These dinner-time diatribes should bring on warm and fuzzy memories, but I think they might be the reason I never instituted this ritual in my own home, choosing instead to eat in front of the television, but that's a subject for another book.

Mealtime moments won't be miserable moments on the Dog Diet. Mealtimes are fun and an opportunity to slow down, prepare an appealing repast, socialize and be creative. I've never been a fantastic cook, although my abilities in the kitchen improved somewhat over the years to the point that I was able to prepare a meal by following a recipe if I needed to, and I could serve takeout in such an artful way you'd never suspect it was anything but straight from my stovetop. I had every gadget and gizmo necessary to prepare all the many concoctions that my endless diets required. George Foreman, Jack LaLanne, Richard Simmons, Bill Phillips—all these guys and their culinary contraptions cycled through my kitchen. It wasn't until Sadie put me through her food mill though, that I got a grip on the enjoyment and pleasure that mealtime and cooking could bring.

Think of eating as a scheduled activity for your day, and make it one of importance. Cook with friends, but be sure to chop vegetables only with people you trust in close proximity with knives. Your life in the kitchen and a relationship with your stove and refrigerator is not over. Although I never did get the message in the *Joy of Cooking* book, I know the joy of eating, and while I was continually trying to deny this on other diets, thanks to Sadie's gift to me of the Dog Diet, joy and food are no longer at war in my kitchen. Here are some great ways to make mealtime into a most enjoyable part, not only of your day, but of your life, your relationships, your health and the bond you share with your dog.

1. If you're having an informal dinner with a date or friends, it's fun to allow everyone to make their own salad. You can create a small salad bar on a kitchen island or counter.

2. Presentation is important. If you've ever been to one of Roy Yamaguchi's restaurants, you know what I mean. Everything I've ever had at one of his restaurants is a work of art. Simple creative touches at home can add pizzazz to your dishes. There are dozens of items on the Dog Diet food lists that can be used as garnishes. Try olives on a little wedge of cheese, a slice of mango with grapefruit on a lettuce leaf or a sprig of fresh cilantro on an orange section.

3. What you eat *on* is also important. I'm not advocating that you run out and buy an overpriced set of china. Bright-colored dishes such as Fiestaware are great for morning meals. Invest in a nice set of larger-size salad bowls for lunch, and a set of dishes that represent something you like for dinner. I have dishes with beach themes and flatware bearing a nautical theme.

4. Coffee mugs can help set the tone for your morning. I have coffee mugs from the places I've traveled. Some mornings you'll find me sipping coffee on Kiawah Island or Aruba; others I'm in New York or any of a number of memorable places I've been. These also make great conversation starters when you have guests.

5. Use place mats to set the mood for your meal. Place mats are very affordable and come in unending themes and materials. Having a tropical breakfast? How about a rattan place mat?

Formal dinner or hoping to impress a date? Something elegant in a dark color or one that matches your dress. Lunch with the girls? Brightly colored woven place mats with different colored cloth napkins are great. And don't forget to have a variety of napkin rings.

6. Where you eat is important. Most mornings, I eat breakfast in my kitchen at the wooden island. Lunch is usually in my sunny comfort corner, and I try to eat all my dinners in the dining room. (My sister Bonnie was kind enough to use her decorating skills to transform my dining room from a dark, dismal, denlike room that I seldom used into a bright seaside café. The project was very inexpensive and a fun sister experience. Fun, because she did most of the work!) If you don't like your eating spaces . . . change them!

7. Make each mealtime moment a mindful one. Take time to experience the taste and texture of your food: the crisp crunch of a fall apple with cinnamon for dessert, the smooth feel on your tongue of the pureed vegetable sauce on the chicken or the many different tastes from the salad.

8. Music is a nice touch during meal preparation and while you eat. Rare is the restaurant that doesn't have background music that attempts to impart ambiance to your dining experience. You deserve no less at home.

9. Candles should be a prominent part of dinner. Candlelight imparts softness to the atmosphere and signifies that something special is going on. Even when eating alone, light a candle. You'll eat more slowly and enjoy the meal.

10. Enter into eating. Yes, after all the years of concentrating on what should or should not be eaten, memorizing the vital statistics of dozens of food items, craving, sneaking and bingeing, I finally learned to enjoy eating and make dining a delightful, not a depressing, event. It took a four-legged canine to put me through an extreme food makeover, but she freed me from seeing food as the culprit in dieting.

11. Realize that a meal is for feeding your hungry body, not your hungry heart. Channel your thoughts in a positive direction while eating, visualizing the food as building blocks for your new, lighter body.

12. Cook for your dog as well as for yourself. Turns out the vet's mandate on no human food for Sadie wasn't exactly necessary. Your healthy diet is also good for your dog, although I still haven't got Sadie chomping down green salads.

13. Don't rush preparing or eating. I tied myself into so many time guidelines with previous diet restrictions that it was like reordering my life every time a diet plan failed. Make mealtimes at your convenience. Not only will you avoid a chopped finger or two by preparing your meal leisurely, it builds anticipation for eating your creation.

14. Mealtime mantras are pleasant thoughts you indulge in while eating. This is probably the best aid to digestion you'll ever discover. Replay the blessings of your day as you enjoy the fruits of your labors . . . vegetables and proteins too!

There are hundreds of other moments in our fast-paced days, and we can't remember each and every one of them. That's why it's so important to hold on to the ones we make special and to make as many moments as wonderful as we can. I think of my "dog moments," such as when Sadie jumps on my lap for a hug. I think of my "bath moment" when all my muscles relax in the warm, fragrant water that now actually covers my entire body since I'm thinner and can fill the bathtub to within a few inches from the top without displacing water on the floor when I get in. Then my reverie is broken by the splash of a tennis ball in the water and the dancing eyes of my diet-dog peering at me. Oh well, nothing lasts forever, not bubble baths, or great dinners, or vacations or life for that matter. It's all in the moments—they last forever in memory, but we have to put them there.

I've learned from Sadie to allow some slack in the leashes that govern my life, and in doing so, I've quit choking myself with unnecessary anxiety while experiencing unexpected joys.

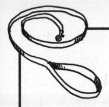

Dog Diet
DISCOVERIES

1. Dogs live in, not out of, the moment. So should you.

2. Magic moments are monumental—treasure them.

3. Save souvenirs for your soul each day you live in the moment.

4. Happiness doesn't happen—it's chosen.

5. Tomorrow's special memories are from an ordinary today.

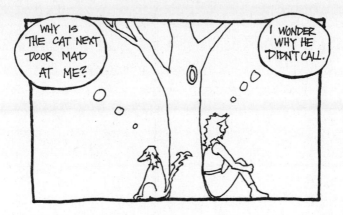

CHAPTER NINE

What's Eating You?

(Dogs don't hold grudges)

*T*he Dog Diet was a new way of life for me. Every day brought some new insight, and remarkably, every week brought yet more weight loss. My eating and physical activities were all structured around Sadie's schedule and needs, but I loved it. After all, I'd never lost this much weight without it costing me money or suffering for each and every pound. I was no longer experiencing many of the mental roadblocks that had plagued me for years and driven me to seek solace in food. My mood in general was better, and while being in better physical shape had a lot to do with it, I was wondering what else had happened to cause this welcome change. I'd seen ads before of people who were hypnotized to lose weight, so I knew my mind had to have something to do with it. My bad moods and failures had been influenced a great deal by my obsessive eating habits, which, of course, increased my weight or kept it at an unacceptable plateau.

Think of all the miserable moods you've suffered just because of clothes that are too tight! If you do manage to squeeze into something that fit when you were ten pounds lighter, it's almost an intolerable experience. Jacket buttons get loose, zippers break, metal hooks and eyes become useless as they are stretched out flat, and the wrinkles at the waist of your skirt are so ingrained it takes more than one trip to the dry cleaner to remove them. Clothes aren't like shoes that will stretch by the end of the day. No sir, the standard pair of tight pants just seems to shrink as the day goes on, but, of course, the large Italian lunch might have something to do with that. No matter how tight something was, if I was determined to wear it, I'd squeeze into it if at all possible. Then I'd vow to myself that I wouldn't eat all day just to be able to wear the outfit, but by lunchtime my resolve had vanished. So I'd spend the afternoon in pain and fear that the seams of my pants were going to split.

I'd compounded this dilemma one day when I locked myself out of my house. My law clerk Season and I had been to a local Mexican restaurant for a very large lunch. I was so uncomfortable afterward that I decided to go home and put on something larger to wear. When I got home, I discovered that I had locked myself out of the house, as well as the backyard.

I called Season at the office and asked her to come over to help me. Somehow, she boosted me over the back privacy fence, and I was then able to unlock the gate and let her in. We were lucky to find a ladder left by my home's previous owner and to find a downstairs window that was unlocked. Fortunately, it was not one that was wired to the security system because it was a very small powder room window that no normal-size thug or burglar could ever slip through, even if their entire body was greased in oil. Here I was in clothes that made it difficult for me to breathe, stuffed with burritos, tacos and corn chips, attempting to ooze myself through it.

Halfway through, I just sucked in my breath and miraculously scraped through and was at last in the house. I was so mad. Mad at myself, mad at Season for suggesting the stupid restaurant in the first place and really mad that I had not only split the seams of my pants, but ripped the arms of the blouse as well. I stuffed the entire outfit into the trash.

Nothing is more irritating in the morning than grabbing a favorite suit or pair of pants only to realize they won't fit, and no amount of breath-holding, lying flat on the bed to zip it or wearing the jacket without a blouse underneath will squeeze you into it. (I'd actually had a few close calls with that jacket-sans-top routine. My office would get hot, and I'd forget that I had nothing on under the jacket and start to remove it.) The end result is that you have to toss the too-small clothes on the bed and frantically search for something larger. That's why I have black pants in three different sizes, and most of my friends also have various-size clothes in their closets. Talk about getting your day off on the wrong foot or, in this case, the wrong size!

This can serve as a deterrent to after-work snacking if you go straight to your bedroom when you get home instead of to the kitchen. There they are: the discarded garments lying on your bed in the afternoon sun reminding you that the chocolate and pizza went straight to your waistline, and you might never be able to wear these treasured togs again. I know because I've returned home from work to face as many as a dozen outfits that had to be rejected that morning. The sight of them had been enough in the past to make me forgo a raid on the refrigerator and bolt straight out the front door for a fast walk that would hopefully decrease my size by the following morning.

During my depressing winter, I was more likely than not to just shove them off the bed, onto the floor, and then kick them underneath the bed. I had no intention of making any radical changes that might enable me to wear them anytime soon. I didn't care if I ever wore them again at that point. Most days, I'd just turn on the gas fireplace in my bedroom, curl up on the rug in front of it with my down comforter and take a nap.

Now that I'd been losing weight thanks to Sadie, struggling with clothes that didn't fit was rare. It seemed, too, that I always ate more than I should have on those now-rare days that had started in a foul mood when the clothes I wanted to wear didn't fit. I realized that my overall good attitude had a lot to do with this weight-loss wonderland I'd not only entered, but been able to actually stay in long enough to see tangible results. Looking back not just at the depressing winter, but all my adult life, I realized I'd held a lot of grudges—against the world and against myself. My discontent and my weight obsession were not just about what I'd been eating, but what had been eating me.

I was not the best dog mom for quite some time after Sadie came to live with me. I just had no experience in dog care and hadn't been prepared for her dropping into my life. Expectant parents spend nine months reading books and talking to other parents. For me, one day I was living in my self-indulgent world, and the next I was trying the best I could to meet the needs and demands of a strange new dog. As much as I hate to admit it, I was downright selfish. Here are a few of the numerous reasons Sadie could've become resentful and held a grudge against me:

1. I returned her to PetSmart because she kept me up that first night.
2. I left her alone for very long periods of time.
3. Initially, I only fed her dry dog food.
4. I was embarrassed at her enthusiastic greetings when I'd return to the car.
5. I tried more than once to leave her in the backyard alone.
6. I tried to make her sleep in the basement.
7. I wouldn't let her on the couch.
8. I gave her too many baths.
9. I talked on the phone too much.
10. I'd forget she was home waiting for me and went somewhere after work.

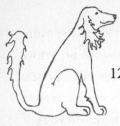

11. I'd curse at other drivers when she was in the car, which scared her.

12. I'd throw her chews away before she was done with them.

13. I'd shut her in the garage accidentally.

14. I was careless and tramped on her tail more than once.

15. I often didn't give her enough sniffing-time during our walks.

16. On the rare occasions I ate out, I didn't always bring home leftovers . . . for her.

17. I tried to control hair loss by using the vacuum cleaner on her.

18. I tried to make her believe I was eating something she wouldn't like.

19. I'd make her wait too long to go out and pee when I was reading my e-mail.

20. I took too long to give her a name.

21. I had dozens of pairs of shoes, but she only had one collar and leash.

22. I insisted on running the lint roller over her before bed.

23. I brushed her ears too much.

24. I wouldn't let her lick the flavored lip gloss off my lips.

And the list could be even longer, but none of these indiscretions seemed to matter to her. She loved me in spite of my many failings. If a person did the human equivalent of any of these to me, I would've been really resentful. Think about it. Have you ever had a male friend rush you through window-shopping? This is the same thing to a dog when you jerk the leash while she's sniffing. How about giving someone a great box of chocolate and they don't open it and give you a piece? In my book, not sharing chocolate is reason to hold a *huge* grudge. In fact, I never give chocolate to someone if I have the slightest premonition that person is not going to share it with me. And how about being on a road trip with someone who, determined to break the time record, refuses to stop at roadside rests? These are all serious infractions of human decency and they can (and do) cause major resentments.

But this little dog just carried on her activities seemingly oblivious to my shortcomings until I was totally smitten with her and voluntarily corrected my bad behavior. Her cheerful demeanor and enthusiasm for just being with me made me slink away in shame over how I'd been acting. Since Sadie was willing to forgive and forget my daily trespasses, I began to examine my own stubborn habit of hanging on to things that bothered me. Every morning she got up with a clean slate, and even as the day went on and little problems would occur, she was quick to wag her tail, lick my face, and the infraction was immediately erased from her memory.

I looked at some of the major reasons I was always stressed out and why I used this stress for an excuse to eat. During this retrospection, I realized how very unimportant my missteps and character flaws were in Sadie's world. If I stepped on her tail, she'd jump up on me and want to be petted. When I threw her chews away, she'd grab her rope toy as a substitute. Sadie's world was a kinder, gentler place— one that I wanted to become a part of. Maybe if I started giving myself the benefit of a doubt and a break now and then, I'd be able to do it for those around me as well. My stresses were no different than most people's: money, love, success, family, and the one shared by millions, weight. None of these seemed very important to Sadie. As long as there was food and water in her bowls, she got taken out for walks, and I was there to be her family, she seemed quite content. The fact that people's usual stresses were nothing in the eyes of my dog brought me to a new attitude. It was time to lighten up my mind now that my body was heading in that direction. I wanted to see how it would be to look at my life with a new perspective: Sadie's. I'd spent so much time worrying about everything, including what I was eating, that now it was time to take a good look at what was eating me.

Dogs and Forgiveness

The day I went to get Sadie after returning her to PetSmart was a turning point in my life. I just didn't know it at that time. My secretary yelled after me as I left the office, "You know they really shouldn't let you adopt a dog." She was probably right. I was the typical type A personality and a lawyer to boot. As a profession, lawyers are unforgiving, seeking retribution in the form of legal remedies, usually as money, often actually trying to get blood out of stones. I'd bet this was not the profile the pet adoption people had for prospective pet parents. And I had already betrayed this little creature by callously dumping her back at PetSmart the day before.

But there she was in Betty's car looking out the window, and

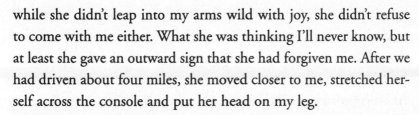

while she didn't leap into my arms wild with joy, she didn't refuse to come with me either. What she was thinking I'll never know, but at least she gave an outward sign that she had forgiven me. After we had driven about four miles, she moved closer to me, stretched herself across the console and put her head on my leg.

She was a smart dog, not holding a grudge against me for my unthinking and foolish decision to return her. She decided not to bite the hand that was going to feed her, something I'd failed to learn in the many disputes I'd been involved in. So if Sadie could forgive me for this most egregious act, then I needed to start forgiving people for much lesser missteps, and myself as well, for the dumb things I did—like switching dry cleaners every time a piece of clothing didn't come back pressed to perfection. And let me tell you, in my town there just aren't that many dry cleaners, so I'd hope they'd forgotten my tirade by the time I made the rounds of them all and had to start at the beginning again. I held grudges for stupid things and harbored these bad feelings for unreasonable time periods—like when I didn't talk to one of my sisters for over a year because she'd forwarded an e-mail to another sister who had promptly gotten miffed at me for the content of the e-mail. I also nursed resentments about things I considered more serious, like not making *Law Review* in law school or feeling slighted by people when they were most likely only busy. I held on to things like this, letting them gnaw at me while I just ate on, trying to cover it all up by comforting myself with food. Viewing things from Sadie's point, these things seemed very insignificant. Not once did I see her run to her bowl and gobble up all the food in response to something I'd done to her. Of course, she did routinely scarf down all the food in her bowl in order to get something of what I was eating, but she was an equal opportunity eater; emotion played no part in it. As she frolicked around my house, she was the epitome of "live and let live," and it was time for me to do so as well.

Three months after I adopted Sadie, I won a fabulous trip—a dream vacation aboard a private catamaran sailing for seven days in the Caribbean, including a private chef on board and dinners at four famous restaurants *and* I could take someone. What a decision. Sure, there was always Rodney, who now was quite attached to Sadie and helped me out with her care if I had to be out of town on business. There was also my mom who would most likely enjoy it, and there were a few girlfriends vying to be the one to go. Instead, I called the sister I hadn't spoken to for all that time and asked her if she remembered why we weren't speaking. She was speechless for a moment. Yes, she did remember, but you know what? It didn't matter anymore. I had heard she was going through a really depressing time, and I was so grateful to be finished with feeling bad that I asked her to be my guest. I was just beginning to learn to let go.

My sister came to visit me that summer and talk about the trip. And while she was here, she used her talents to redecorate the downstairs of my house. I have a beautiful seaside café motif for my previously dark and dull dining room that I never would have conceived on my own. That fall we went on the trip and had a magical time. Sadie taught me not to hold on to hurts, but to let go and not to let them eat at me. Consequently, my life felt lighter, and my mind didn't tell my body it needed the comfort from food anymore.

Dogs and the Pack

I'm from a big family, and there's always someone who's not speaking to someone else, usually for some trivial reason. These squabbles and grudges aren't even confined to my siblings and parents. No sir, we force all the unfortunate people who married into this crazy family to get involved as well. From brothers-in-law to nieces, everyone is fair game. When we get miffed, we let everyone know it, and the person who actually caused the perceived injury gets ignored. In my case, when I was involved in one of these standoffs, it was reason enough to eat everything in sight. During weekends with more than one such skirmish going on, I've gained as much as six pounds eating my way through my perceived hurt and anger.

One of my family's favorite phrases seems to be "remember when," and the memory that follows is not usually warm and fuzzy. Nope, we hold grudges dating back as far as we can remember. "Remember when," I'd tell my sister Amy, "you ruined that leather jacket of mine when we were in high school?" Well, we were having this conversation after we'd both been out of school for more than two decades.

"Remember when," she asked me as we strolled the beach at Kiawah Island under a brilliant star-filled sky, "you embarrassed me and Terry (her husband) when we fixed you up on that date with Bill?" I sure did remember. They'd brought a guy along with them whose jeans were about four inches above his white socks, and his hair was wet, and they expected me to spend the day with him . . . cheerfully. Well, I went along, but not willingly, and I certainly wasn't pleasant company for anyone, including my date, who could have passed for Pee-Wee Herman. (Though, I'm not sure even Sadie would expect me to forget that my sister fixed me up with a Pee-Wee Herman look-alike!) On that same moonlit walk I was reminded of the time I'd shut her cat Patches in the dryer and turned it on, and I asked her to recall when she sold her pony to me for twenty-five cents because she wanted to get penny candy at the nearby country store. It went on and on, from brother to brother, Mom to me, me to a sister-in-law. Something was always eating at me due to one family conflict or another.

I took Sadie to meet my family the summer after I'd adopted her. This was her first trip of any length in the car with me, and it was a disaster. She slobbered the entire trip, threw up at the first gas station I stopped at and in general was a miserable mess. The lady at the gas station had watched as I frantically grabbed every paper towel available at the gas pumps and tried to clean up the car. I had forgotten they have speakers at self-service pumps as I grumbled my way through this ordeal. When I went in to pay, she said, "What happened? Did your little dog get sick?" I told her "no," because I was embarrassed to have been seen wiping up dog vomit and realized she'd probably heard the recriminations I'd heaped on Sadie over this and myself for giving her a dog biscuit before leaving home even though I'd been told not to. I made a lame excuse about spilling a breakfast shake in the car, but I knew she wasn't buying it. "Give her some Dramamine and she'll be okay," she called after me as I left the store. That's a big help now, I thought. I had four more hours ahead of me in a car smelling of regurgitated Milk-Bones. I guess as a dog parent you haven't lived until your dog has thrown up in your car.

By the time we got to my parent's house, I was exhausted, my car was a mess, and my nerves were stretched tight. Trust me, this is not a good condition to arrive in for a visit with my family. Home visits demand the calmest of demeanors and maybe a prescription tranquilizer or two.

Sadie was overjoyed to have the car finally come to a stop and jumped out. Much to my surprise, many members of my family were out in the yard, a welcoming committee of sorts, to meet my new dog. They'd been so taken aback when I told them about Sadie, and then that I had returned her, that I don't think they really believed she existed. She greeted my dad with a puppy version of vicious protective barks but loved my mom immediately. This was unusual. Dogs were always smitten with my dad, and Mom never really liked them. My nieces and nephews overwhelmed her, but she was curious about them and happy to have so much attention. I was happy to dump her off on all these new caretakers and make a hasty trip to the car wash to try and salvage some of my car's usual pristine condition. When I returned, Sadie was overjoyed to see me as usual, and Dad reported that she had whined and seemed lost without me.

I watched Sadie as she cavorted happily in all the confusion. She simply accepted everyone as they were and soon made up with my dad. Jazzie, my parents' sheltie, wasn't happy to see another dog getting all this attention. Sadie, however, was pleased to have her company and tried over and over again to play with her.

Sadie had no prejudgments of anyone in my family (despite what I'd told her as we drove up there) or the other dog for that matter. She was enjoying the attention and playfully swatted at Jazzie. I watched my dad interact with her and noticed how kind he was and how he exuded joy watching her run for her ball and eat the little treats he was slipping to her. I observed my mom giving her a pat or two when no one was looking, and when someone was watching, she made a comment or two about Sadie being spoiled. I caught them sitting on the back porch together, though, in the swing that Mom didn't even allow Jazzie on. Sadie wriggled up to my brothers, my nieces and nephews, and even let her curiosity bring her very close to the big hunting dogs in their cages.

Since I have no children, this was the closest my parents would ever get to a grandchild from me, so I was happy they liked her and she liked them. Sadie ran through the fields and slept on the back porch in Jazzie's crate. It was a wonderful few days of relaxation and fellowship. No "remember whens" and no hurt feelings of any kind. Sadie brought out the best in all of us.

On my way back to Charleston, I thought over what had made this visit so different and pleasant from so many in the past. I looked at Sadie sleeping peacefully on the seat next to me. I had taken the gas station lady's advice, and after consulting with my vet, picked up some Dramamine. Sadie snored every once in a while, but I was so relieved that there was no

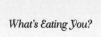

slobbering or worse. She had made the visit such a nice experience, and if I had anything to do with it, all future visits would include her. I was determined that even if there was a misunderstanding or a quarrelsome memory brought up at these get-togethers, I would always make a point to leave in this state of mind.

Membership in families isn't chosen, and although you can elect not to communicate with them, you can never really leave them, and after seeing them through Sadie's eyes, I realized I wouldn't want to anyway. Hey, if I'd have known that it could be this simple, I'd have gotten a dog a long time ago!

Dogs and Success

The question most often asked at business meetings, conferences, cocktail parties and *always* at happy hours is: "What do you do?" Over the years, my answer to this question has changed. I've done or been many different things. From teaching school to being part-owner of a restaurant to being a model at a boat show, my experiences in the employment arena are diverse. I'd learned to work hard at an early age and paid my way through college with many different jobs, including being most definitely the worst waitress to ever spill food on a customer. Diners who had the misfortune to be seated in my station had no idea what they were in for.

Becoming a lawyer was my lifelong dream and was emblazoned as my goal under my senior yearbook photo. After accomplishing it, I was proud to answer the "what do you do" question and respond that I was an attorney. That is until I realized almost every single person I told either had a bad experience with a lawyer, knew someone that had a bad experience with a lawyer or wanted free legal advice. I've suffered through enough lawyer horror stories at social gatherings to last the rest of my life. To my knowledge Sadie had no experience with lawyers, nor had any of her littermates, and this was refreshing.

By nature, lawyers are tense people driven to succeed, and they ruthlessly expect perfection from everyone but demand it from themselves. I was no different. Since graduating from law school, I was out there in the race to stay ahead, make money and win cases. And I had done pretty well, but during the winter of my discontent, I felt all used up and no longer able or wanting to keep going. There was a television show about a guy who ran his law office out of a bowling alley, and I envied this loony lawyer. I longed for my restaurateur days where I could perhaps have a booth in the corner from which to run my practice while having anything and everything on the menu, as well as the inventory of the bar available to me with a slight signal to the nearest server.

After Sadie arrived and as we grew closer, I hated to go to the office because I didn't want to leave her. Sadie was unaware of what I did to support us. She just hated my leaving, and when she did come to my office, she had no idea how self-important all of us were. She'd run up and down the hall of my office spreading rawhide chews along her path, oblivious to the pompous air we believed our office was infused with. She'd sleep under my desk, not at all swept away by the fact that her mom was making a seven-figure settlement over the phone or sending a sheriff's deputy out to serve a lawsuit on an errant taxpayer. Nope, she might just as well be in the break room of a sweatshop—just so long as I was there. I'd received more rewarding looks from Sadie for scratching her stomach than I'd ever gotten from my colleagues for a tricky litigation strategy I'd spent a long weekend developing. The legal world meant nothing to her even though it enabled her to take more than her share of trips to PetSmart for treats. Of course, she didn't get to go to work with me every day, but I'd often pick her up and take her in after a late afternoon hearing, and she was always with me on those long evenings and weekends that are requisite for all lawyers clawing their way through the legal labyrinth of purported success.

Most of the people in my office liked her, or at least they tolerated her, except for the day one of the other female lawyers remarked that it was a good thing a certain person wasn't in the office because that person was allergic to dogs. This was news to me, and being the protective mom I'd become, not to mention an argumentative lawyer, I replied, "Yeah, well, I'm allergic to kids, and she brings them in here."

Having Sadie in the office had never been a problem, but here we were, two female lawyers engaging in this argumentative repartee. I realized how stupid and unimportant it was and let it go. After all, I was catching up with the supermoms in my office—I had more photos of Sadie on my desk and shelves than any of them had of their kids or husbands. And from the complaining I overheard about toilet training kids, Sadie'd been a lot easier to housebreak.

I realized I didn't want my profession to define who I was, and it didn't even come close to exemplifying the qualities I wanted to be known for. I began taking the lawyer thing a lot more lightly after Sadie's appearance in my life. After all, I doubt many dogs discuss what their human parents do, let alone care how much money they make. What was success anyway? My "successful self" had spent a miserable winter where nothing I accomplished was able to bring me the smallest amount of consolation. Now, the happiest days were often the ones where I did the least. I wasn't getting lazy; I was learning how to be happy, which should be the end result of success anyway. Sadie made me realize that what I *did* wasn't who I *was*. Achievement wasn't what made me happy and kept me interested in staying in the game of life. I began using a different kind of gauge to measure whether I felt successful or not—measured in moments, not material accomplishments.

A successful day for Sadie was one where she received several stomach scratches and caught her ball most of the times it was bounced in the air for her. It was a day that wasn't raining. Sadie had a successful experience when she got to lie on the couch with me or eat lunch in the backyard with me. Success to her was getting me to give her a portion of my food or a Frosty Paws ice-cream treat before bed. Success was a day she got to spend with me from morning until night. Knowing how much she appreciated that made my day successful too.

I let go of the grudges associated with my profession. It didn't matter that I hadn't been the lawyer who'd successfully sued McDonald's because their coffee was too hot, or gotten to wear the Tigger suit while successfully defending Walt Disney. It was now irrelevant to my life to strive for perfection constantly or be on the lookout for someone who would get ahead of me. I was only worried about Sadie getting too far ahead of me as we went on our daily walks. I became grateful for what I had, not what I wanted to be. My little dog taught me that success is in the heart, not in a paycheck, a title or a framed certificate on the wall. It's not that firm handshake from opposing counsel after you've won your case or a move to a larger office with a window. It's that wriggle-infused greeting at the end of the day, that lick on your face when you return to the car and that high-speed tail thumping the mattress when you open your eyes in the morning.

Dogs and Weight

Just like a trip to my own doctor, a trip to the vet for Sadie always began with getting weighed. Sadie's first vet had a scale in the waiting room. It was a large stainless steel platform that the dog was expected to stand on. Even though Sadie watched dog after dog step up or be placed on this scale, she refused to get on or stay on when I put her there.

"You can get on and hold her, then put her on the floor, get back on by yourself, and we'll subtract the difference," the vet's assistant instructed me. *Was she out of her mind?* Not only would she know how much I weighed, the benches were filled with animals and people who would also know, as the weight was displayed in large, red, digital numbers on the wall monitor. One particularly slim woman who was closest to the scale was watching closely as this little episode evolved. She had an equally trim, smug-looking cat on her lap, and I couldn't give them the satisfaction of seeing my humiliation when the numbers were splashed across the screen. I refused to do it, despite the pleadings of the vet's assistant. Sadie seemed to share my reluctance at having her weight become public knowledge and refused to stay on the platform long enough for it to be calculated. Very frustrated, the vet's assistant just placed us in a treatment room deciding to let Dr. Paul deal with us.

When the vet entered the room, Sadie was so eager to greet him, he never even consulted the note I'm sure was written in her chart about not being weighed. He played with her, performed the examination, gave me some advice and we were out of there. I knew, however, that we wouldn't be that lucky the next time.

Our next encounter with weight was at her new vet, who, believe it or not, we didn't switch to merely over the public scale situation. Sadie developed a problem that necessitated transfer to a clinic with more experience with her problem. So off we went to the new veterinarian, who weighed dogs somewhere in the back without needing my assistance. What a relief that was. He did want me to monitor her weight at home, though, and instructed me to determine her weight the same way the girl at the other office had explained. This was fine with me. The weighing would take place in the privacy of my own house, and all I had to do was the math and then report Sadie's weight back to them, not mine.

As Sadie was expected to gain some weight, once a week I'd pick her up and get on the scale. If it was more than it had been the week before, I was happy assuming that the extra weight was on Sadie, and most of the time when I verified this, I was right.

But, like many of us, Sadie hated being weighed. In fact she hated it so much that, at last, I ended my silly obsession with the scale. For years I had believed that in order to lose weight I had to get weighed every day. Now I was getting on the scale once a week and continuing to lose weight.

The end of the scale regimen was also the demise of all the other regimented weight-control rituals. I stopped keeping meticulous charts of my daily or twice daily weigh-ins. Gone were the journals recording every morsel of food that went into my mouth and the composition of each bite as to calories, fat and so on. No longer did I write down every physical activity I performed in order to justify the amount of food I'd consumed. Nope, things were simpler. I wasn't consumed with the numbers on the scale anymore—until I called a hotel to see if I could bring Sadie along on a business trip.

The hotel advertised that they allowed dogs for a onetime $25 registration fee. What they didn't say—until I called to actually make the reservation—was that the dog had to weigh fifteen pounds or less. Well, hey, I'd been lying about my weight for years now. I mean, how many of us actually weigh what's printed on our driver's licenses? And I have yet to have anyone point out any discrepancy to me. So, I figured, what was five pounds, especially to a dog? I gladly agreed to fill out the registration form they faxed to me. This turned out to be quite an ordeal.

Questions such as how old is the dog, which I translated to mean is she old enough to be housebroken or too old to still be

housebroken? How many hotels care how old their guests are anyway? Is she used to being alone? Hey, she was coming with me, why
would she be alone? They must have experienced guests who parked
their dogs in the room and headed straight for the hotel lounge, but
I had no such plans. And then, the deal-breaker question, how
much does she weigh?

With the same breezy nonchalance I used when I lied about my
own weight, I boldly wrote down "fifteen pounds" and didn't give it
a second thought until I received the confirmation a few days before
we were supposed to go. It clearly stated that the fifteen-pound
weight limit was strictly enforced and a violation of it could result in
having our reservation canceled. Horrified, I envisioned a scale sitting right in the middle of the hotel lobby, like at the vet's office. I
could see being asked to weigh Sadie and, when she refused, being
asked to go through the same ritual I'd refused to perform at the
vet's. The lobby would most likely be filled with businessmen with
nothing better to do than observe my humiliation. No way was I
going to take this chance. Maybe it was easier for a human to dis-
guise a ten-pound weight discrepancy, but with dogs I was
unsure and felt I'd be better off not going.

When I called to cancel, I was flustered and meant
only to say that something had come up and I
needed to change my plans. But the entire ordeal was
so unnerving that I blurted out that I couldn't make it
because we weighed too much. There was a long
silence and then I was given a cancellation number, but
no invitation to call them back.

Dogs and Dating

If there was ever an area of my life where grudges were paramount, it was dating. After years of dating Rodney, he hadn't wanted to get married. So I made the decision to date someone from my past in hope of a future. Well, that too was a fiasco, and it was from this heartbreaking romance that I was reeling when I adopted Sadie. Since then, I've met many women who got dogs after ending a marriage or long-term dating relationship. It turns out that dogs are the best medicine for broken hearts, and Sadie certainly was far nicer to me on a consistent basis than most men I'd known. During our first few months together, I told Sadie all about the guy who had broken my heart, and about Rodney, who was endearing himself to her more and more. I warned her, "Don't count on him, Sadie. He's nice, but he can't make a commitment and will just want to see you when it's convenient for him." I told her that sooner or later she'd have to take the step I'd taken when I decided to date someone else. That clearly had not been a wise decision. After all, wasn't she here to try and put my heart back together?

Truth is, I was harboring a great deal of resentment toward Rodney. Had things been different between us, I wouldn't have gone through this horrendous romantic devastation with someone else. But Sadie didn't have these feelings about him, didn't pay any attention to my directives and continued to shower him with great affection every time she saw him. I began calling him her "dad" and for a confirmed bachelor, he really seemed to enjoy this.

During one of our consultations with Dr. Abbott at Virginia Tech, I commented that one of Sadie's mannerisms was just like her dad's. Dr. Abbott was quite surprised and said it was great that I knew who her dad was and how unusual that was for a shelter dog. Everyone in the room got a great laugh when I explained it was her human dad.

I finally decided to get back in the dating game. This brought on an entirely new set of decisions to make. It's always difficult to find your way when dating someone new, but add a dog to the mix and it's downright confusing. Like, when was I supposed to introduce a prospective partner to Sadie? I decided to do it early on because if she didn't like him, it wouldn't matter if I did. How could I justify leaving her alone in the evenings when she was alone all day while I was at work? I limited my early dating trials to dinner-only enterprises, which involved a minimal amount of time, but they were also welcome respites because, initially, I was still going through my food battles at home with Sadie.

First there was the banker I'd met when his bank refused to cash one of my client's checks through the drive-through window. Outraged, I parked my car, grabbed Sadie and entered the bank, demanding to have the check cashed. I had no idea that a Mr. Possibly Right was standing to the side enjoying the scene. After a quick apology from the customer relations manager, I was introduced to this man. In the usual manner, we exchanged business cards, and he called me.

He and Sadie got along quite well, but now I am sure it was only because of the carob-coated biscuits he brought her and all the leftovers I eventually began sharing with her. He played with her and even got down on the floor to wrestle with her. I heard him tell her as I lingered outside the entry hall, "I really like your mom." This clinched it for me and for Sadie. But I soon discovered that he liked the moms of lots of other dogs too, and that was the end of that.

Next, I began dating a doctor. My mother was ecstatic. We had a few extravagant dinners and some minimally interesting conversation. I found myself doing the same thing to him that people did to me when they belligerently asked for free legal advice. I asked him for some weight-loss tips, which had nothing to do with his area of practice. His suggestion for quick weight loss was a fast of sorts: eat only 400 calories a day of anything I wanted. I never knew if he was serious about this or just wanting to avoid any more $100 dinner tabs but still continue to see me. Despite my mom's pleadings to "give him a chance," I dumped him. Four hundred calories a day! I'm sure I've eaten more than that from my bedside chocolate stash before my feet ever hit the floor in the morning.

After one more dating debacle with yet another banker that a friend of mine had fixed me up with, I threw in the towel. Sadie was much better company than any of these men, and if it hadn't been for the great dinners, none of them would have lasted the short time they did anyway. I'd come home from these evenings and tell Sadie all about them. I also let go of them with no ill feelings.

So Sadie and I began spending more time with Rodney than I'd ever spent with him while we'd been dating. He'd come over to "see the dog." He'd bring dinner by without asking and call to say he'd like to join us for her last walk of the night. He took on the official role of drying her ears after baths, and her vet said she never got ear infections because they were so clean and well cared for. He'd go to PetSmart with us and offer to pay for her goodies. The three of us ate lunches in a nearby park, cruised around town in Rodney's vintage convertible, fell asleep watching movies. As the first football season approached after Sadie's adoption, he got her a little yellow football. I knew he was hooked.

Sadie also had assimilated some of my traits as well. She lost her toys almost daily. She'd search frantically all over the house for Mr. Cheeseburger or her rope chew. I placed a small cardboard box in the living room, and each evening before bed we made a game of gathering all the toys and placing them in the box. By the time I left for work the next morning, they were scattered to the four corners of the house, and when I returned for lunch, I'd watch her resume the search for them. Sometimes she'd realize they were in the backyard and paw at the door and at me, wanting me to go out with her to find them. Sadie didn't rest until they were all gathered back together, and her jubilation was uncontained when she'd discover one of the missing toys in an obscure corner of the backyard.

Maybe Sadie had something here. Maybe everything I felt was missing from my life when I went searching for a new romance had been right here in my backyard, or more accurately, across the street. I mean, it wasn't like I'd had a grand time out on the dating circuit. And it was difficult to date anybody new anyway with Rodney popping in unexpectedly all the time to see Sadie. I realized that neither the sad nor resentful feelings concerning love were occupying my time anymore. I felt love again, completely and unconditionally, for Sadie, and, who knew, maybe I could feel the same for someone of my own species thanks to learning to let go.

Want to feel lighter and weigh less? Then take a look beyond what you are eating to what's eating you. Have family problems? Think how they appear to others, including your dog, and you might see them differently. Dissatisfied with your career? Make a move or find things there to be grateful for. Looking for love? Get a dog, and you'll be too busy to miss having a boyfriend, and ultimately you'll learn what love is really all about. Do you not eat at a restaurant you used to love because you are certain the bad service was a personal slight against you? Get over it; go have a great dinner. How about the neighbors? Not on speaking terms? Take them some flowers from your yard or fresh tomatoes from your garden. Worked too many hours this week? Go get a massage or a pedicure.

As for me, I know there will always be irritating things in life, and I know, even with Sadie's lighthearted spirit as a constant reminder, I won't change overnight, nor will I become a completely different person. I do know now, though, that heavy thoughts made me a heavy person. That heavy body weight is very often directly connected to our mental weight. I know that I'll still get mad at the neighbors for loud music at two in the morning and at my bank when they make a mistake with my account. At restaurants, I still send dishes back that don't suit me, have squabbles with my siblings and call myself stupid when I make a dumb mistake. But Sadie gave me the benefit of the doubt, and I've learned to give it to myself and extend it to those around me. I've also quit biting the people I love, and I've quit growling about things long after they're over. I have also let go of striving for perfection—in body or behavior.

I no longer have a perfectly clean house, nor do I have the perfect job, the perfect boyfriend or the perfect body. Even with the new sweeper and dust buster, dog hair has overtaken my hardwood floors that once upon a time I wouldn't allow anyone to walk on with shoes. I'm still waiting to win one of those multimillion-dollar lawsuits that will be reported on every television channel, but as a lawyer, I at least find my job challenging, and it does allow me to afford some pretty nice dog toys and vet bills. My body is in good shape, and my appetite has shrunk because my heart isn't hungry all the time. And as for boyfriends, well, we'll see. Even though there aren't any weddings on the horizon, Rodney is still there for Sadie and me, steady and sweet, with a sense of humor that keeps me smiling. He's still the quintessential bachelor, but after all, he's Sadie's dad, so we have to try to work things out for the sake of our dog-daughter.

Come to think of it, I have a *perfectly* wonderful life and I thank Sadie for it. When she turned my world upside down, I was able to see things from a different perspective. The principles of the Dog Diet have brought things into perspective for me, and I'm no longer tripping over my leash in a quest for perfection. Calling my new way of life the Dog Diet kept something familiar in my life—the word "diet," but it's not a diet like anything I've ever known before. Unlike all the other diets I've followed, it doesn't drive me constantly toward perfection—and you know what? I'm glad.

I've come to believe that Sadie is the perfect companion, friend and confident. With true dog-parent pride, I also think that she is just about the most perfect dog on earth. Even so, I've learned a huge lesson about perfection from a most unforeseen source.

It had been almost a year since our first visit to Virginia Tech and the infamous french fry incident. We were again traveling the same road home from the hospital—happy that Sadie's test results were perfect and that her heart problems were now a thing of the past.

The road sign said that McDonald's was just two miles ahead. As we got closer to the interchange, Sadie sat up on the seat and began sniffing the air. The closer we got, the more she sniffed. I had been so nervous about her tests that I hadn't eaten lunch and was hungry, but I'd learned in the past year not to eat in the car, and we were only about an hour from Charleston and our own kitchen. Besides, I didn't eat while driving anymore, and Sadie might get sick if I allowed her to eat without taking Dramamine. We didn't need junk food, right? I may have forgotten a lot of things in the past year, but I still had a pretty good memory of how one of those McDonald's fish sandwiches tasted along with a vanilla milkshake. I'd never actually seen a square fish, but it was delicious—wherever it came from.

Twenty minutes later we're back on the road to home. Two cheeseburgers, one fish sandwich, two vanilla milkshakes and a shared apple pie later, Sadie and I had become partners in a food crime. I certainly wasn't going to tell anyone, and I doubted she would either, so we cruised along smug in our secret indulgence.

I pulled up to the tollbooth to pay the fee, and, as usual, Sadie, who has been the recipient of dog biscuits from countless bank tellers and gas station attendants, stuck her head out the window, ready for a treat.

"Hey, what's that all over your little dog's mouth?" the attendant asked warily as he ducked back into his booth. It seems Sadie was not as good at keeping food secrets as I'd thought. For the rest of the trip she lay on the seat contentedly licking the mooched dog treat crumbs from her lips while trying to remove the evidence of our food felony in the form of dried vanilla milkshake which had stuck to her nose and whiskers.

As for me, I didn't get any milkshake on my face, because I've had much more practice than Sadie at surreptitious eating, but I sure have refreshed my memory of that fish sandwich. Okay, I also had one of the cheeseburgers. But hey, we've gotten through a lot of things this past year together— but we never said we'd gotten perfect!

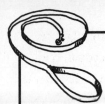

Dog Diet

DISCOVERIES

1. Grudges are like gaining weight in your heart.

2. People shouldn't bite.

3. Give yourself a break, and everyone around you will benefit.

4. Comfort foods make clothes uncomfortable.

5. Success isn't always being the top dog.

6. Sometimes what you're looking for is already in your own backyard.

7. So what if you do get perfect? Then what?

PART THREE

The Dog Diet Plan

Making Your
Salad Box

The Salad Box is the basis for all your Dog Diet meals. Depending on what you choose to put in it for the week, your meal combinations can be endless. This is where I learned to "get one over on Sadie." I had a great stash of good food at my fingertips for consumption at any moment and *none* of it was interesting to her. It was fantastic to just stand at the kitchen island and eat from the box with abandon. Soon I actually started enjoying the taste of the raw vegetables and lettuces, and when I added chocolate mint to the contents, it was almost heaven! Here are the steps for preparing your very own Salad Box.

Make preparing the Salad Box a fun activity. Shop for the ingredients when you can take your time. Look first for what's in season. Cary Neff, the former chef at Miraval Spa in Tucson, Arizona, advocates building your entire meal on seasonal vegetables, and the freshest and smallest are the best.

Equipment

1. A storage container large enough to hold salad ingredients and vegetables for a week. It should be one that opens quietly—just in case your dog decides to like salad and fresh vegetables! I use a Rubbermaid Seal 'n Saver two-gallon size. It has a rubber seal and keeps salad ingredients fresh for the whole week.
2. Cutting board.
3. Sharp knives.
4. Mandoline. This is optional, but having equipment in your kitchen that looks like only a professional chef can operate it adds credibility to the times when you try to pass off takeout for your own cooking to a prospective boyfriend. Mandolines are very easy to use and are great for slicing vegetables into thin slices, or even crinkled slices, and you can get slicing done in record time.
5. Stainless steel strainer.
6. A blender. If you have a full-size blender, great! If you use a blender mostly for smoothies, Hamilton Beach makes a very affordable personal-size blender that is perfect for one smoothie, and the blender container even comes with a lid for those times when you want a healthy meal or snack on the run.
7. Wire whisk. These come in various sizes.
8. Food grinder or food processor.
9. A grater (for vegetables and to grate fresh Parmesan).
10. An electric mixer.

Procedure

Plan your grocery shopping for Sunday afternoon, when you can take your time preparing the box for your week ahead. Fix a nice glass of rosemary water and take your time—enjoy the moment!

1. Wash all the vegetables and lettuces and allow them to drain in the strainer.
2. Pat dry as much as possible with paper towels.
3. Place the lettuces at one end in the box without cutting or tearing. You won't develop any of those ugly brown edges this way, and you can shred, tear or cut it when making your salads.
4. Slice the cucumbers, carrots, onions, squash and whatever else you've selected for the week.
5. Add the two vegetable selections. For example, one week I'll have broccoli and fresh baby yellow squash and different choices for the next week.
6. Pop everything into the box, cover with a paper towel.
7. Make sure the lid seals tightly and place it in the refrigerator UPSIDE DOWN. This removes the remaining water from the vegetables.

There you have it. All set for the week. For each meal you'll make a salad, select a vegetable and add some protein.

Dog Diet
Shopping List

$\mathcal{B}$efore you go to the store, take a minute or two to determine how much food you'll need for the week. If you're like me, wasting food is never a problem, but extra food means extra eating and thus extra pounds.

You won't find a lot of packaged diet foods on this list, however in the "Time-Saving Tips" section, you will see some excellent choices for when you are in a time crunch. I've also included good cheese. You don't have to use a lot to have the great flavor of cheese, and best of all, you don't have to pretend to like the fat-free stuff that tastes like the plastic it's packaged in.

However, the basis of the Dog Diet is the Salad Box, and the more variety you fit into the box for the week, the more variety of meals you can make in a moment. The secret to success with this shopping list is not to buy *anything* that will sabotage your diet. So if you stress out over something and eat four bowls of lettuce—no problem.

If it looks like the week will be full of situations that might cause food overload, leave special, but dangerous-in-large-quantity, items like the blue cheese crumbles at the store! Free yourself from the temptations and food challenges of the past. Shop only for Dog Diet approved items. Gone are the days of calculating percentages and ratios of fat to protein to carbs to overeating.

Five Easy Shopping Rules:

1. Eat *before* shopping!
A hungry shopper is an impulsive shopper.
2. Stay on the perimeter of the store as much as possible, but avoid the deli and the bakery— there are treacherous traps located there in the form of bagels, chocolate brownies and cheesecake, just to name a few.

3. Ignore the tabloids with tempting quick-fix diets.

4. Stick to your list, and don't linger over choices. Save the real shopping time for shoes.

5. Make it your goal to only shop once a week.

Buy what's in season first. Baby vegetables are the best and the season for fresh produce is short. Buy only enough for one week.

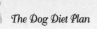

Your Basic Salad Box Should Include

Carrots, shredded   Onions *(red)*

Celery   Peppers *(green, red or yellow)*

Cucumbers   2 seasonal vegetables of your

Lettuce, any variety   choice *(see Fresh Vegetables list)*

Fresh Vegetables

*Freeze fresh
mint and
rosemary in
ice cubes to
make water
extraordinary!*

Beets   Potatoes

Broccoli   Radishes

Cabbage *(green and red)* Sprouts

Cauliflower   Sugar snap peas, in pod

Corn   Tomatoes

Green beans   Turnips

Green onions   Yams

Jicama   Yellow squash

Mushrooms   Zucchini

Fresh Fruit

Apples   Pears

Avocado   Plums

Blueberries   Raspberries

Grapefruit/oranges   Strawberries

Kiwi fruit   Watermelon

Mangoes

I have no idea how to really use lemongrass, but it gives a great flavor to many things, chicken in particular, smells great and makes me feel like I know how to cook.

Fresh Herbs

Basil

Chives

Cilantro

Dill

Garlic

Ginger

Lemongrass

Marjoram

Mint

Oregano

Rosemary

Tarragon

Thyme

Protein

Canadian bacon

Chicken breasts

Eggs

Fish *(such as yellow fin tuna, tilapia, orange roughy, sea bass)*

Lean chicken sausages

Lean pork chops

Salmon

Scallops *(nonprocessed are best)*

Shrimp

Tuna

Turkey

Dairy

Blue cheese crumbles *(the ONLY cheese Sadie won't beg for)*

Cottage cheese

Fresh Parmesan

Good-quality cheese *(Havarti and Stilton are two of my favorites)*

A *small* package!

Black Refried Beans:
I use El Rio brand, but any kind is fine. I'm not sure how you would even begin to make your own refried beans, but I'm not willing to learn when these are just great!

Ricotta *(use the part-skim, low-fat variety of any brand)*
Skim milk
Soy milk and soy cream for coffee
Yogurt *(Dannon Light 'n Fit Carb Control with Fiber is a great choice. Plus it comes in the cutest little four-packs!)*

Grains and Legumes

Black bean dip
Black or kidney beans
Black refried beans
Brown or wild rice
Cereal (*I like Kashi*)
Couscous
Garbanzos
Whole wheat *(Nutri-Grain)* waffles
Whole wheat bread or English muffins
Whole wheat orzo
Whole wheat pasta
Whole wheat tortillas

**Desert Pepper Brand
Black Bean Dip:**
This can be used for bean burritos and in recipes. It has only 25 calories for 2 tablespoons and NO FAT . . . plus, it's enough to make you lick your lips, and Sadie has NO interest in it!

**La Tortilla Brand
Whole Wheat Tortillas:**
These tortillas are not only delicious, they are loaded with fiber. They come in four flavors: Original Whole Wheat, Green Onion, Tomato Basil and Garlic Herb.

Condiments

Almonds or walnuts, slivered

Desert Pepper Trading Co.
   Peach Mango Salsa

Dried cranberries

Flaxseed

Hot sauce

Ketchup

Lemon/lime juice

Low-fat mayonnaise

Mustard (*all varieties*)

Olive oil

Olives (*all varieties*)

Peanut butter

Pickles

Pine nuts

Pumpkin seeds

Lemon and Lime Juice:
*I use the ones that come in the
imitation plastic lemons and limes
when I need more than a squeeze
or two of juice. They're convenient,
and, hey, if you don't mind carrying
one around in your purse, they're
great to add to bottled water
throughout the day.*

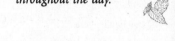

Salsa: *There are those
Martha Stewart types out there
who actually make salsa, but I learned
my lesson the hard way here.
My one attempt to make salsa required
four different telephone calls to the
hospital emergency room. I didn't have
any rubber gloves to wear for handling
the habanera peppers, and my hands
were on fire. I fell asleep that night
clutching two wet washcloths filled
with ice. Now any salsa that comes
in a jar is fine with me.*

Sauerkraut: *It makes a
good almost-zero-calorie snack
that your dog won't be the least bit
interested in, and come to think of it,
you won't be crazy about it either,
but hey . . . if you're hungry and
trying to keep your weight down . . .
why not? There's really nothing
quite like a large bowl of sauerkraut
to take away cravings and
curb your appetite.*

Roasted Italian peppers

Rosie's Sweet or Hot Red Pepper Spread

Salad Dressings: Annie's Naturals (*anniesnaturals.com*) are my favorite, except for the ones I make myself *(see recipes)*. Here are some great choices from Annie's:

Low-fat Gingerly Vinaigrette

Organic Asian Sesame

Organic Green Garlic

Organic Papaya Poppy Seed

Roasted Red Pepper

Shiitake Sesame

Tuscany Italian

Salsa

Sauerkraut

Sunflower seeds

Dried Spices

Basil

Blackened redfish spice

Cajun spice

Cayenne pepper

Curry

Cinnamon

Dill

Garlic-pepper blend

Ground ginger

Italian seasoning

Jerk spice

Lemon-pepper seasoning

Marjoram

McCormick's Salad Supreme
(*Great for pasta salad*)

Mrs. Dash

Nutmeg (*Grate it into your coffee*)

Old Bay

Oregano

Paprika

Paul Prudhomme Blackened
Seasoning

Red pepper flakes

Rosemary

Sea salt

Sesame seeds

Tarragon

Thyme

Tony Chachere's Original
  Creole Seasoning

White pepper

Whole black pepper

Desserts

Blue Bunny Fudge Bars: They can't be beat. Well, actually they
  can—with some deep chocolate, real fudge ice cream—but I
  have to remember I gave all my larger-size jeans away, so I stick
  to the Blue Bunnies!

Sugar-free Jell-O and pudding mixes

Whipped cream in the can: It's only fifteen calories (hard to break
  the habit). Sadie loves this and she gets a squirt or two.

Beverages

Make your beverages calorie free.

7-Up Plus—in the new "in" color pink

Aqua Cal flavored water with added calcium

Calorie-free ginger ale

Coffee

Green tea

Fuze Diet White Tea *(Pomegranate)*

Perrier or other sparkling water

Sugar-free Red Bull

Necessary Luxuries and Scents for Mealtime Moments and More

At least one set of nice dishes and glassware

Candles for the table

Chocolate! Very dark chocolate in single-serving pieces. Okay, if you can't find it that way, just one candy bar, but it has to last the entire week!

Flowers

Fresh mint and rosemary to serve in water

Lavender Hydrolat Naturopathica (*Miraval Spa, Arizona*)

Mint Gymnasia Quenching Cream and Buffing Grains (*Bath Bloomers, Charleston, South Carolina*)

Mochaccino Body Scrub (*Ajune Spa, New York*)

Place mats and cloth napkins

Pomegranate Wash (*Origins*)

Relaxing music CDs (*I like Yanni or anything New Age.*)

Wake-Up Rosemary (*Essential Elements*)

Sadie's Shopping List

Breath Buster Biscuits

Chicken Soup for the Dog Lover's Soul Dog Food (*dry and canned*)

Crazy Dog Piña Colada Scented Shampoo

Dentley's Chew Rites for both home and office

Dogswell Treats (*Mellow Mutt and Happy Heart*)

Frosty Paws

Kong *(when frozen with peanut butter, I'm in heaven.)*

Little Cesar Select Dinners, all varieties.

L'Oreal Kids Tangle Tamer, for her ears (*Sweet Pear Scent*)

Neon-colored tennis balls

Science Diet Nature's Best, chicken flavor

Second Wind Energy Snacks, for squirrel chasing

Toothpaste (*chicken or peanut butter flavor*)

Tropiclean Papaya Plus Shampoo

Very LONG leash, for squirrel chasing

Seven-Day
Dog Diet Meal Plan

*Y*our shopping list will remain basically the same each week, and the variety of the meals depends solely on your imagination. From the same stock of healthy, mainly odorless, quiet foods, you can make any number of different variations. This seven-day guide is only that—a guide. Unlike other diets, you don't have to eat certain things on specific days or at set times.

There are five simple things to remember:

1. Breakfast is not a synonym for fried eggs. Last night's leftovers can make a great breakfast.

2. Cook enough protein for dinner to be used with the next day's lunch.

3. It's all about the presentation. Take your time, and make your meals as beautiful as you want them to taste!

4. Use your imagination—combine ingredients in unusual ways.

5. Just about anything tastes better with whipped cream on it. According to Sadie, even dog food!

Recipes for many of the selections in the "Seven-Day Dog Diet Meal Plan" can be found in the "Dog Diet Recipes" section.

Sunday

Breakfast

Whole wheat (Nutri-Grain) waffles topped with
vanilla yogurt and fresh strawberries

Iced green tea with fresh mint

Midmorning Snack
Granny Smith apples and cheese

Lunch

Chicken Frittata

Arugula Endive Salad with lemon, olive oil
and Parmesan dressing

Midafternoon Snack
Sliced tomato topped with cottage cheese

Dinner

Roasted Chicken

Grilled Asparagus and Red Peppers

Salad with roasted red pepper dressing

Sliced mango and cottage cheese

Monday

Breakfast

Cereal and milk

Fruit

Midmorning Snack

Yogurt with sliced almonds

Lunch

Arugula Chicken Wraps

Midafternoon Snack

Cottage cheese with dried cranberries

Dinner

Grilled Shrimp with Avocado

Grilled Asparagus

Yams with butter and brown sugar

Toasted whole wheat bread

Chocolate pudding with whipped cream

Tuesday

Breakfast

Bean burrito with salsa

Fruit

Midmorning Snack

Cottage cheese with olives

Lunch

Black Bean and Shrimp Green Salad

Sliced fruit

Cheese wedge

Midafternoon Snack

Grapefruit with cinnamon

Dinner

Grilled Blackened Salmon

Corn with salsa

Side salad

Apple Yogurt (Fit & Fiber Dannon)

Wednesday

Breakfast
Egg Salad Muffins

Fruit

Midmorning Snack

Fruit and olives

Lunch
Green salad with
cold Blackened Salmon

Fruit Pizza

Midafternoon Snack

Chocolate Java Ricotta Supreme

Dinner
Whole Wheat Pasta with Olive Oil, Fresh Herbs
and Grilled Chicken

Jell-O and whipped cream

Thursday

Breakfast
Yogurt and strawberries

Whole wheat tortilla with butter and cinnamon

Fruit

Midmorning Snack
Cucumber, cherry tomatoes and cottage cheese

Lunch
Cold Pasta Salad

Sliced tomato with cottage cheese

Dinner
Grilled vegetable plate

Egg white omelet

Salad

Fantastic Peach Sundae

Friday

Breakfast
Sadie Smoothie

Fruit

Midmorning Snack

Cottage cheese and mango salsa

Lunch
Bean burrito

Salad

Fruit

Midafternoon Snack

Deviled eggs with endive

Dinner
Roasted Chicken Stuffed with Rice

Vegetable

Salad

Chocolate Java Ricotta Supreme

Saturday

Breakfast

Chive and cherry tomato omelet

Warm whole wheat tortillas

Citrus fruit

Midmorning Snack

Sliced Granny Smith apples with cinnamon

Cheese wedge

Lunch

Tomato Stuffed with Chicken Salad

Cold Brown Rice Medley

Green salad

Midafternoon Snack

Yogurt and cottage cheese blend

Dinner

Reservations!

Schedule for a Dog Diet Day

6:00 a.m. Rise and Stretch

Imitate your dog here. Watch how she stretches and do your own version as described in chapter 6. Dogs seem to have the right idea about how to start the morning! Turn on the music and get moving. Make the bed. Get dressed. Move to the beat in a few rounds of Dog Dancing. Bound down the stairs for that morning walk!

7:00–8:00 a.m. Morning Walk

(If you don't have this much time, remember anything is better than nothing!)

8–8:30 a.m. Breakfast

YOURS

½ cup cottage cheese
1 cup fresh strawberries
1 small whole wheat tortilla,
warmed and spread with light
butter and cinnamon

YOUR DOG'S

1 Tbs. cottage cheese
Chicken Soup for The Soul
dog food (dry and canned,
mixed)

Both: Take your vitamins; give your dog any medications, vitamins and so on.

Big serving of cold fresh water!

Quick session of Dogercise . . . take your pick from chapter 6.

SNACK FOR WORK	**TREAT FOR CRATE**
One apple, cut in sections and sprinkled with cinnamon	Breath Buster Biscuit
1 part-skim mozzarella cheese stick	

Off to work.

12:00 p.m. Home For Lunch

12:15–12:45 Noontime Walk

It's very easy to get in one mile. Walk fifteen minutes away from the house and back. De-stress from the morning's work details. Be as happy to be with your dog as she is to be with you!

Lunch

YOURS	**YOUR DOG'S**
Large bowl of salad greens and vegetables from your Salad Box	Cold brown rice mixed into food
Sliced cold chicken breast	
Yogurt	

A few sessions of catch and Dogercise and back to work you go.

Midafternoon Beverage

Enjoy a cup of green tea; I like the Republic of Tea flavored ones. Wild Berry Plum is my favorite.

Keep a nice glass in your office for water. It doesn't have to be Waterford, but a heavy, clear glass to keep water in through the day is excellent. And you can freeze ice cubes with mint in them to keep in your office refrigerator to add a little taste of luxury! Exciting!

Home from Work

Don't delay the walk; pass the kitchen and go!

Change clothes, get your dog ready and get out the door. I take a sugar-free Red Bull Energy Drink for me and Sadie's collapsible water bowl.

We do two miles and then stop for a short rest and both have a drink of water. We look at the river, pause to think over the day, watch birds and boats and other walkers. And then we walk the two miles back, ready for dinner and a relaxing evening.

Dinner

YOURS	YOUR DOG'S
Black bean/chicken burrito with salsa ½ cup cottage cheese with mango salsa	Cold brown rice mixed into dog food, with some finely chopped vegetables from the Salad Box

Late-Night Snack

YOURS   **YOUR DOG'S**
Sugar-free chocolate pudding with   Frosty Paws
 whipped cream

End of Day

Think back over the good things that happened today. Give your dog a hug. Rub some peppermint cream on your feet; have a great night's sleep. Your day was as good as any dreams.

Dog Diet Recipes

(Or directions purporting to be!)

$\mathcal{T}$he word "recipe" automatically makes us think that some type of cooking will be involved. Don't be so sure with the Dog Diet recipes. Remember, it's all about making your life lighter: more fun, less stressful and more enjoyable. So in the spirit of that, and knowing how dangerous it is to the survival of a healthy weight to spend too much time in the kitchen, these directions for creating meals are short, easy, fun and not to be taken too seriously!

Not Your Typical Recipe Rules

1. *You can substitute anything you want. Change chicken for fish or fish for eggs. Switch spices to suit your own tastes.*
2. *The portion sizes are at the discretion of your dog: what you can eat before she discovers it. Most of the recipes are for four servings, allowing you to freeze leftovers for later or refrigerate for a repeat meal later that week.*

3. *Measurements are not exact.*
4. *Experimentation is expected and encouraged.*
5. *Sometimes opening packages or jars quietly is work enough.*

Recipe Index

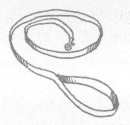

Arugula Chicken Wraps

Finely chop 1 cup of cooked chicken and mix with
1 cup of shredded arugula.

Add chopped onions, green chilies,
2 Tbs. of low-fat mayonnaise and 1 tsp. of tarragon.

Stir everything together and mix thoroughly.

Take one whole wheat tortilla and spread with
a light layer of low-fat mayonnaise.

Spread the chicken mixture on the tortilla.

Add greens from the Salad Box.

Roll tightly. Slice in half.

Another version of this, if you need to impress someone,
say, with afternoon tea . . . *(Hey, you MIGHT just have
afternoon tea!)* is to spread the mixture on individual
leaves of endive. Place a layer of greens from your Salad Box
on an elegant plate and arrange the endive boats.
Add sliced avocado, grape tomatoes and sliced almonds.
Drizzle Lemon Olive Oil Dressing over everything.

Yummmmm!

Arugula Endive Salad with Lemon Olive Oil Dressing

Wash and drain arugula and endive.

Arrange artfully on plate or bowl.

Grind fresh pepper on top.

Prepare Lemon Olive Oil Dressing (see page 254).

Slowly drizzle dressing over salad.

Grate fresh Parmesan over the top.

Eat and enjoy!

Black Bean and Shrimp Green Salad

Remove a portion of lettuces and other vegetables from the Salad Box.

Arrange in a large bowl.

Open and drain 1 can of black beans.

Clean and devein previously cooked shrimp.

Add beans and shrimp to the mixed salad.

Put some salsa in a small glass bowl.

Add olive oil, lime juice and some crushed garlic.

Whisk thoroughly and pour onto salad.

Toss.

Delicious!

Chicken Frittata

(This is a great brunch entrée!)
Mix ½ cup diced chicken, 4 egg whites, and
¼ cup each of diced potatoes,
onions and green peppers.
Cook in a nonstick skillet.
Sprinkle with fresh chives.

Chicken Meat Loaf

2 boneless chicken breasts *(or ground chicken)*
½ cup chopped green pepper
¼ cup chopped onions
Selected spices
Black ground pepper
1 egg
¼ cup bread crumbs

Using a food grinder, grind the first six ingredients
together and mix thoroughly in a large bowl.
Add bread crumbs to hold the mixture together.
Mold into a loaf pan and bake at 350° for 45 minutes.
Save some meatloaf for sandwiches.

Tip

One useful way to maximize the effort involved in making chicken meat loaf is to make a sufficient quantity to freeze and use for more than one meal.

- *Mold into meatballs and serve with whole wheat spaghetti.*
- *Mold into chicken patties.*
- *Use in chili.*
- *Make stuffed green peppers.*
- *Make cabbage rolls.*

Chocolate Java Ricotta Supreme

Empty one 8-ounce container of part-skim ricotta into a glass mixing bowl.

Add 2 Tbs. of instant coffee and 1 Tbs. of miniature Hershey's Dark Chocolate Chips.

Add sugar or any other sweetener to taste.

Mix together, divide in two and place into small dessert dishes.

Chill for at least an hour.

Serve with a squirt of whipped cream.

You'll think it's crème brûlée!
(If you really have a good imagination!)

Cold Brown Rice Medley

Combine 1 cup of cooked wild or brown rice with
chopped celery, red onion, green chilies,
chopped arugula, sliced almonds and corn.

Add 3 Tbs. of Annie's Natural Shiitake Sesame Dressing.

Mix thoroughly.

The leftovers will keep for about a week in the refrigerator.

Cold Pasta Salad

Using the leftover pasta from a previous meal, sprinkle
generously with McCormick's Salad Supreme.

Finely chop cucumbers, red onions, olives and green pepper.

Add whole grape tomatoes.

Toss all the vegetables and the pasta together.

Use low-fat Italian dressing to taste and mix with the salad.

Egg Salad Muffins

Cut up the whites of 2 hard-boiled eggs.

In a small glass bowl, mix the egg whites with
chopped celery, onions, green chilies and chopped olives.

Add 2 Tbs. of coarse brown mustard.

Cut 1 whole wheat muffin in half and toast lightly.

Place 1 piece of Canadian bacon on each half.

Divide the egg salad in half and place on the muffins.

Eat both or save one for later!

Fantastic Peach Sundae

Remove the lid of one container
of Peach Yogurt.

Add a squirt or two of whipped cream!

Fruit Pizza

*(WARNING: I only make this when I am having
company, and I limit myself to one slice!)*

Spread one 18-ounce package of sugar-free cookie dough
(your choice) on a round pizza pan and follow
package directions for baking.

In a bowl, with an electric mixer, whip
an 8-ounce package of cream cheese with ½ cup of sugar
and 1 Tbs. of lime juice.

Select any number of fruits, slice them and set aside.

After cookie dough is cooked and cooled,
spread cream cheese mixture over the cookie pizza.

Arrange the fruit and press down into the cream cheese.

Chill in refrigerator.

This is the ONLY Pizza that your dog will not beg for!

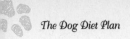

Grilled Asparagus and Red Peppers

Wash asparagus and peppers.

Slice the peppers into strips about a half inch wide.

Place vegetables in a sealable container.

Drizzle with olive oil and spices.

Place lid on and shake until thoroughly coated.

Place vegetables in a pan and broil until desired doneness.

They can also be cooked on the outdoor grill.

Grilled Blackened Salmon

Wash the salmon and pat dry with a paper towel.

Sprinkle blackened seasoning
(I like Paul Prudhomme brand) on both sides.

Place under broiler.

Cook as well done as desired.

Grilled Shrimp with Avocado

Clean, peel and devein shrimp.
I like larger shrimp, but any size will do.

Put the shrimp in a small glass bowl.

In another bowl, mix together olive oil,
Tony Cachere's Cajun Spice mix (Old Bay also works great),
coarse black pepper and sea salt.

Pour mixture over the shrimp and mix well.

Place on a nonstick surface under the broiler for
about 3 minutes each side.

Peel and slice an avocado and squirt with lemon juice.

Arrange on a plate and serve!

Lemon Olive Oil Dressing

In a small bowl (I like the little glass ones because
they make me feel like I know what I'm doing!),
whisk together 2 Tbs. of olive oil, lemon juice
and fresh-ground pepper and sea salt.

(Those little wire whisks are perfect for this part of the preparation.)

Omelets
(A Word About Omelets)

Egg white omelets are easy to make,
and your choice for ingredients is unlimited.

The general procedure is to chop all desired
ingredients and place in a bowl.

Separate the egg yolks from the whites
(4 egg whites make a nice-size portion).

Mix everything together and cook thoroughly.

Garnish with salsa, black beans, cilantro
or cheese as desired.

Roasted Chicken

Pull back the skin on the breast of one whole roasting chicken
and insert garlic cloves and other spices as desired.

Rub lemon juice and pepper onto the outside of the chicken.

Cook chicken in oven according to package directions.
*(This will be the protein base for several meals
and you can also freeze it.)*

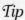

Tip

I take the entire chicken apart when it has cooled.
I place the chicken into containers and store in the refrigerator.
To satisfy Sadie, I chop up some chicken and
pour some of the broth over her dog food.
I then prepare a second storage container of
chicken for her and place in the fridge.

Roasted Chicken Stuffed with Rice

In a small glass bowl
(Trust me on this glass bowl thing—you, too,
will feel like Julia Child!),
mix 1 cup of cooked wild rice with chopped onions
and celery, spices,
1 egg and bread crumbs.

Stuff the chicken with the rice mixture.

Cook the chicken according to package instructions.

Sadie Smoothie

After years of chugging down bland drinks in an effort to lose weight, I swore no more liquid meals. BUT . . . you can make great smoothies with unlimited flavors, and they taste good. The best part is, your dog won't want them, so you can sip away and enjoy. This is one of my favorites and is named after Sadie, even though she hasn't had one lick!

Fill blender about halfway with ice cubes.
Crush.

Add 8 ounces of skim milk, ½ cup cold coffee,
1 Tbs. natural peanut butter and one container of
vanilla yogurt.

Bottoms up!

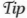

Tip

*A fruit variation of this smoothie is
an easy and quick breakfast, as well as
a great way to use up fruit that is very ripe.*

Tomato Stuffed with Chicken Salad

Cut cold cooked chicken into cubes.
Mix with chopped scallion, cilantro, green chilies
and celery.

Stir in low-fat mayonnaise.

Scoop out one medium-size tomato and
stuff the tomato with chicken salad.

Tuna

Solid white albacore tuna packed in springwater is an excellent
lunch when you add it to your salad. You can share some with your
dog; just mix some in her food. She'll love it!

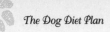

Whole Wheat Pasta with Olive Oil, Fresh Herbs and Grilled Chicken

Place a mixture of Italian seasoning, fresh Parmesan
and crushed garlic into a freezer bag.

Place 1 pounded-thin chicken breast into the bag and shake well.

Grill the chicken and set aside.

Cook 4 servings of whole wheat pasta and drain.

Place half of the pasta into a large bowl.

Remove a small amount of the pasta to share with your dog.

Chop fresh rosemary and crush garlic.

Mix the herbs with olive oil using your whisk.

Cut the chicken breast in half and place one half
in the refrigerator for another meal.

Cut the remaining chicken into strips and mix into pasta.

Pour the olive oil/herb mixture over the pasta and toss together.

Grate fresh Parmesan over the pasta before eating.

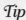

Tip

*There are many flavored olive oils on the market
and many variations for this dish are possible.
I also like portobello mushroom–flavored olive oil
mixed with crushed garlic and finely chopped
shiitake mushrooms and scallions.*

Let your imagination be your guide.

Time-Saving Tips

Being crunched for time as well as worrying about crunching your food within earshot of your dog can be daunting. Here are some easy solutions for saving time. I don't recommend them as a regular routine. After all, living in the moment means enjoying the moment, not trying to rush through it. But, if using a shortcut is necessary, take time to enjoy something else that day.

1. Use packages of premixed salads. There's a wide variety out there to choose from. You can open them and pop the contents into your Salad Box along with the vegetables.
2. You can also get a bag of prewashed broccoli and carrots for your vegetables.
3. Too busy to cook? Lean Cuisine dinners are acceptable (in a crunch) and the spa line is excellent. The microwave still attracts Sadie and the meals smell delicious, but I've solved the problem by letting her lick the container and leaving a

few bites for her. She sits patiently waiting for her portion, and I can eat without interruption.

4. Make bean burritos ahead and store in the fridge. You can add salsas, lettuce and so on to them in a jiff, and they are good to go!

5. Buy the containers of cottage cheese that have fruit packaged with them. These are great for traveling as well.

6. Keep fresh herbs frozen in your freezer. While great chefs use only the freshest herbs, the culinary-challenged like me hardly know the difference.

7. Buy diet green tea in bottles and you can just remove the cap and enjoy. No boiling water, which on some days can be quite challenging.

8. Cook enough rice or pasta for the entire week and store in the refrigerator. It can be eaten cold or warmed up.

9. You can usually find a free cruet in the supermarket if you buy an Italian dressing mix. This can be used to make your own salad dressing to keep in the fridge. Or save an empty mustard jar and the lid.

10. Cook enough protein for the entire week. A turkey breast cooked in a slow cooker is an excellent solution for a week when you are very busy.

Time-Stretching Tips

We live in a sleep-deprived, multitasking world that offers few moments of respite. Here are ten things you can do to actually make the moment last longer. You probably won't have time for all of them in any given day unless you're incarcerated, but try to do at least one a day. Create a space in time and stretch it to the limit.

1. Brew and drink a cup of tea. Don't gulp it, don't read the paper. Just sip the tea and make it last as long as possible.
2. Take a fifteen-minute nap.
3. Do the crossword puzzle.
4. Buy some flowers and arrange them yourself.
5. Clean out the junk drawer.
6. Take a bubble bath by candlelight.
7. Write a note to someone expressing your appreciation for them.
8. Listen to a CD from start to finish.
9. Brush your dog slowly and thoroughly.
10. Sit silently looking at the stars for fifteen minutes before bed.

Travel Tips for a
Dog Diet Road Trip

*H*ere are some great tips for traveling with your dog and taking your Dog Diet habits on the road with you. A vacation or short trip shouldn't be a time when you abandon all your new good habits.

1. Take along a small cooler with snacks for both of you. Be sure to include:

   • Bottled water
   • Yogurt
   • Fruit
   • Hard-boiled eggs
   • Fresh-cut vegetables

2. Don't forget a water bowl for your dog. The new collapsible ones are great.

3. Keep a supply of plastic spoons, napkins and other items you deem necessary in your car.

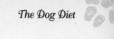

4. Neither of you need to eat while driving. Stop at a roadside rest stop (never along the side of the road) and take a break.

5. It's never a good idea to leave your dog in the car, but if you must for your own very quick bathroom break, make sure you are parked in the shade with windows down a few inches for air, and use a car harness instead of a leash. (Available at *PetSmart.com*)

6. Take Dogercise breaks at rest stops. Indulge in some toss and retrieve with the ball you've brought along. (Keep your dog on a leash at rest areas.) Do some stretching and tug-of-war. Try a few mealtime squats . . . just the thing to loosen up those leg muscles from driving.

7. Fast Food: If you can't make do with your cooler snacks, then fast food from a drive-through will work *if* it's Dog Diet approved. The following fast-food restaurants have items that are acceptable for both you and your dog while traveling. Take advantage of the outdoor dining areas most fast-food restaurants have, or find a nice place under a tree for an impromptu picnic!

   • Wendy's—Grilled chicken sandwich, grilled chicken salad, small plain hamburger, baked potato, side salad.

   • McDonald's—Grilled chicken sandwich or salad, small plain hamburger, fruit salad, any of the new gourmet salads.

   • Subway—Any of the low-cal, low-fat sandwiches are fine and can also be ordered as a salad. One of the small deli sandwiches will work fine for your dog. The wraps are also great here. Sadie and I find the menu at Subway perfect for sharing just about anything. Avoid anything with heavy sauces or spices if you are sharing with your dog. (Remember—they're not that great for you either.)

- Burger King—Vegetable sandwich, grilled chicken sandwich, salads, plain Junior Whopper.
- Taco Bell—The soft chicken taco is your best bet.
- Others—Most fast-food places will have the same type of selections. Use your best judgment. Don't let your appetite guide your selections, just choose foods or the closest substitute to the foods used on your Dog Diet daily menu.

If your dog is like Sadie and wants to eat constantly, but isn't a good traveler, I'd suggest you stick to the snacks from your cooler. There can be a wide variety of humiliating scenes if you try to eat when your dog can't have anything. Sometimes, it really is best to just skip a meal!

Special Tip #1—The Web site www.letsgopets.com has valuable information for traveling with your dog.

Special Tip #2—Sadie and I also look forward to room service at our favorite pet-friendly luxury hotels! Look for your digs at www.petswelcome.com.

EPILOGUE

$\mathcal{A}$s summer turned into fall, the anniversary of when my heart had broken was approaching. By now though, my life had developed a happy rhythm with Sadie that was unbelievably comfortable. I no longer looked back, and I had no regrets; however, I did have some unfinished business waiting silently for me all this time on the third floor of my house.

The day came when I knew that it was time to tackle the dreaded top floor where during my depressing winter I had thrown everything I couldn't deal with. And I mean everything . . . numerous items of clothing that needed mending, boxes from all the Internet junk I'd ordered . . . mail I didn't want to deal with . . . fragments of the fractured romance in the form of letters and items I'd not been able to throw away.

I carried Sadie up the stairs and began the onerous task of sorting through a life I was glad no longer existed. It was a puppy's paradise: things to bite everywhere, papers to chew, mountains of clothes to climb on and burrow under. There it was, among the flyers, boxes, packing foam and clothes whose seams had burst as I had gotten bigger—that package from Harrods, purchased what seemed a lifetime ago. I crawled through the debris and picked it up. Sadie immediately pounced on it as I opened it.

Inside were the carefully packaged Waterford goblets I had purchased for a romantic encounter doomed even before I'd crossed the Atlantic with them. I opened the boxes and carefully removed them from the numerous layers of packing. They were as exquisite as I remembered them, and the late summer sun caught them and splayed little rainbows on the wall. Sadie sat and watched the light show with extreme fascination.

I had been transformed in the preceding months, and these glasses that I'd hidden up here when the very sight of them crushed me no longer had that power. I felt the emptiness where the sadness had once dwelled, and I had more than enough to fill it up with now.

I ran down the stairs leaving Sadie to watch over the glasses as they sat glistening in the sunlight. I returned quickly, running up the stairs with a bottle of Perrier. I poured the sparkling cold water into each glass. One I placed in front of Sadie, and I picked the other one up. It seemed an appropriate time to celebrate . . . the beautiful chime of the elegant crystal echoed loudly on the walls as I clicked my glass against Sadie's, and without the smallest trace of sadness of anything lost, I said, "Here's to us, Sadie."

Sadie stuck her little face right down in the sparkling water and loudly lapped up the bubbles as I drank deeply and swallowed, feeling the effervescent water go down my throat, and as it did, a feeling washed over me that was slightly bittersweet and ever familiar— it was love.

ABOUT THE AUTHOR

*P*atti Lawson is an award-winning author, trial attorney and journalist. She is a frequent contributor to the *Charleston Gazette* and other publications. She writes a column titled "DOGS . . . DIETS . . . DATING," which appears in the *Charleston Sunday Gazette/Mail.* Patti is also an accomplished public speaker and presents seminars to civic and women's groups on a variety of topics. She and Sadie are very involved in fundraising events for shelter dogs. They live in Charleston, West Virginia.

NOTES

NOTES

NOTES